Preventing and Reversing Osteoporosis

Every Woman's Essential Guide

Alan R. Gaby, M.D.

PRIMA HEALTH
A Division of Prima Publishing

PRIMA HEALTH and colophon are registered trademarks of Prima Communications, Inc.

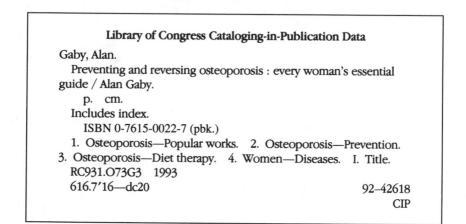

Library of Congress Cataloging-in-Publication Data

Gaby, Alan.
    Preventing and reversing osteoporosis : every woman's essential guide / Alan Gaby.
      p. cm.
    Includes index.
      ISBN 0-7615-0022-7 (pbk.)
      1. Osteoporosis—Popular works. 2. Osteoporosis—Prevention.
    3. Osteoporosis—Diet therapy. 4. Women—Diseases. I. Title.
    RC931.O73G3   1993
    616.7'16—dc20   92-42618
                                            CIP

98 **AA** 10 9 8

Printed in the United States of America

How to Order:

Single copies may be ordered from Prima Publishing, P.O. Box 1260BK, Rocklin, CA 95677; telephone (916) 632-4400. Quantity discounts are also available. On your letterhead, include information concerning the intended use of the books and the number of books you wish to purchase.

Visit us online at www.primahealth.com

Contents

Foreword

A born professor must teach, and with this volume you and I are again the beneficiaries of Alan R. Gaby's research and insight. *Preventing and Reversing Osteoporosis* is the book from which we can learn things that, if past behavior is any indicator, the medical establishment won't "learn" for 20 to 30 more years. Dr. Gaby was told more than once in medical school to "shut up about that mineral and vitamin research stuff, never mind that it's published in medical journals." Luckily for us, he pursued his interest in nutrition and natural medicine. A man who insists on integrity and free scientific inquiry, Dr. Gaby approaches his work with intelligence, energy, enthusiasm, humor, and attention to detail. Whether he is lecturing, treating patients, or writing columns, articles, or books, Dr. Gaby takes pains to ensure that his work is accessible to everyone.

Besides being a gifted teacher, Dr. Gaby is also a talented researcher. His skill is in sifting through vast amounts of research to cull promising early research findings. He then knits these findings into uncannily accurate and useful treatments for problems that still baffle much of medical science.

Dr. Gaby is able to pinpoint successful alternative treatments because he works from a fundamental principle: the body is a whole. He demonstrates in this book that to take care of our bones, we must take care of our whole bodies and our overall health. What's good for the bones is good for the heart, the skin, the breasts, the stomach, and even crucial for future generations. In *Preventing and Reversing Osteoporosis,* Dr. Gaby goes beyond the current calcium craze to a holistic approach to healthy bones.

In taking good nutritional care of our bones (and bodies), we must be concerned not only with the quality of what we eat, but also whether nutrients are digested, assimilated, metabolized, and retained—all of which are discussed here not as incidentals, but as integral aspects of optimal bone (and body) health. Where else can you read about the importance of strontium, vitamin K, and silicon in bone health? Especially all in one place.

Since this book is written in the late twentieth century, a discussion of mineral toxins (lead, cadmium, tin, aluminum) as well as acid rain is relevant and included here.

One of the big "osteoporosis questions" of the last two decades has been the role of estrogen. Dr. Gaby gives estrogen a new perspective, and working again from the "whole body, whole bone" principle, he tells us of research on other hormones that directly affect bone health.

Since *Preventing and Reversing Osteoporosis* will probably be studied with a bit more personal interest by women than by men, Dr. Gaby has done as he always has in teaching and has included a chapter of invaluable information about other women's health problems, including PMS, fibrocystic breast disease, abnormal menses, abnormal PAP smears, endometriosis, yeast infections, menopausal symptoms, and breast cancer.

I first met Alan Gaby when he moved across the country to study with me; he quickly became a friend as well as a student. Now, in the best tradition of scholars everywhere, he has surpassed his teacher in more ways than one.

Preventing and Reversing Osteoporosis is ample evidence.

Jonathan V. Wright, M.D.
Tahoma Clinic, Kent, Washington

Acknowledgments

Jonathan V. Wright, M.D., and Davis Lamson, N.D., for fostering a climate of intellectual curiosity and for helping extend the boundaries of the possible; Michael Murray, N.D., for tirelessly searching the medical literature and sharing with me hundreds of important articles; Fritz Perlberg, for helping me stay motivated and focused; Andi Reese Brady and Melanie Field, for their excellent editing; and the many scientists and doctors whose research made this book possible.

Introduction: Is There Really New Hope?

Osteoporosis is a major cause of suffering and disability among the elderly in America, particularly among elderly women. The progressive thinning of the bones that occurs with aging causes millions of women to suffer painful and disfiguring fractures, sometimes after only minimal physical trauma. Hip fractures are a common reason that elderly individuals end up in nursing homes and are an indirect cause of death for hundreds of thousands of people each year. Fractures of one or more vertebrae in the spinal column turn previously tall, robust, and healthy women into "little old ladies": twisted, frail, and in pain.

Conventional medical opinion is that osteoporosis is a relentless process that cannot be reversed and that the best we can hope for is to slow down the rate of bone loss. So women do things that are supposed to help, while hoping for the best. They faithfully take calcium supplements, do some aerobic exercise, and agonize over whether the benefits of taking estrogen are worth the risks.

Despite these preventive measures, at least 1.2 million women suffer fractures each year as a direct result of osteoporosis. To make matters worse, the number of osteoporotic fractures seems to be increasing. More than twice as many major fractures occur now, compared with thirty years ago, and this difference cannot be explained by the aging of the population. Clearly, there is something wrong with our bone health, something that the medical profession has not been able to do much about.

This book offers new hope in the fight against osteoporosis. It presents exciting new evidence that there is more to preventing bone loss than calcium supplements, estrogen replacement therapy, and exercise. It challenges long-held dogma by arguing that osteoporosis is not only preventable, but can most likely be reversed, as well.

THE MEDICAL ESTABLISHMENT RESISTS NEW IDEAS

It is easy to be cynical, or at least skeptical, about medical writers who promise "new hope." If there really were a new approach to osteoporosis, wouldn't all the star research scientists from the top-notch universities know about it? Evidently not, because scientists with impeccable credentials who have spent their careers studying osteoporosis still say that the best we can do is delay or minimize the damage. How then can someone else come along, claiming that osteoporosis can not only probably be halted in its tracks, but that there is even reason to believe the irreversible can be reversed?

During twenty years of studying medical research and fourteen years of clinical practice, I have learned that many important advances and effective treatments originate outside of the medical mainstream and can take years or even decades to be incorporated into conventional medical wisdom. Classic examples of this "cultural lag" in medicine abound. For instance, when Sir James Lind discovered that British sailors could avoid the ravages of scurvy by eating limes his findings were ignored for fifty years, while hundreds of sailors died needlessly. When Ignaz Semmelweis, an Austrian physician, found that an epidemic of maternal deaths during childbirth could be eliminated if doctors would only wash their hands before delivering babies, he was ridiculed and harshly censured. When Sir Alexander Fleming reported that penicillin, a common mold, could cure pneumonia, his findings were not taken seriously for more than a decade.

Today, despite major advances in communication and information dissemination, the process by which new treatments are incorporated into the medical mainstream is sometimes just as slow as it was centuries ago. A new remedy is more likely to face opposition if it is based on ideas and concepts that do not conform to the prevailing point of view. Specifically, treatments that emphasize lifestyle modifications or administration of nonpatentable, naturally occurring substances are more likely to be ignored than are new drugs or surgical techniques. This bias against natural medicine retards progress, since many of the most valuable treatments available originate from within nature.

About twenty years ago, I became interested in the possibility that dietary modifications, nutritional supplements, and other "natural" remedies could be used as the basis for a new approach to medical care; one that would be safer, more effective, and less expensive than the usual drug and surgery approach. Pioneers such as Linus Pauling, Roger Williams, Carleton Fredericks, and Adele Davis had written about this controversial new concept. They argued that many diseases could be prevented or treated by adjusting the concentration of molecules normally present in the body, such as vitamins, minerals, hormones, and so forth. Although this idea seemed logical, it was alien to prevailing medical dogma. Nevertheless, these writers were able to cite hundreds of references to support their point of view. After investigating most of these references, I decided to incorporate nutritional medicine into my practice. It soon became clear that, for many medical conditions, it is possible to obtain better results than the textbooks and the "experts" say is possible. As a result, my therapeutic imagination, unlike that of other physicians, is not hampered by the "official" medical viewpoint. In other words, if medical dogma holds that a disease is irreversible, I do not necessarily believe that dogma.

REVERSING THE "IRREVERSIBLE"

When I think of "irreversible" disease, I am reminded of the case of a desperately ill seventy-nine-year-old rabbi. After four heart attacks, his badly damaged heart was in the final stages of congestive failure. The previous twelve months, spent mostly in the hospital, had been relentlessly downhill. Like many patients with congestive heart failure, his weight had fallen from his usual 171 pounds to a severely emaciated 113 pounds. His cardiac ejection fraction (the percentage of blood ejected into the circulation with each beat of the heart) was only 19%, barely enough to keep him alive. He was confined to bed and required supplemental oxygen much of the time. To make matters worse, his peripheral circulation had deteriorated so badly that six of his toes had become gangrenous. An angiogram of the extremities showed complete blockage of the femoral-popliteal arteries in each leg, with "poor distal runoff." In other words, whatever small amount of blood was making it to the feet could not be seen on the angiogram. As his condition progressed, even maximal doses of morphine taken every three hours put only a small dent in the severe pain in his toes.

Two independent vascular surgeons felt that immediate amputation of both legs above the knee was necessary. They were convinced that if he did not have the amputations, the bacteria from the gangrenous tissue would enter his bloodstream and kill him within two weeks. Unfortunately, the cardiologists were convinced that the patient's failing heart would not last another month, regardless of what happened to his legs.

The rabbi refused amputation and, instead, called my office to seek one last try with nutritional therapy. I began treating him with intravenous injections of magnesium, B-complex vitamins, and trace minerals, as well as large oral doses of vitamin C, vitamin E, folic acid, and some other nutrients. The results were nothing short of astounding. After six weeks, the pain had improved, the oxygen mask had come off, and the cardiac ejection fraction had increased to 36%. With continued treatment, the gangrenous areas sloughed off, and pink, healthy tissue appeared underneath. The rabbi also began to gain some weight, a turnaround considered impossible by authorities in cardiology. In fact, so certain were the cardiologists that his "cardiac wasting" was irreversible that the rabbi was told to regard any weight gain with alarm; a sign that his lungs were filling up with fluid. But he continued to gain weight over the next twelve months—34 pounds of healthy tissue and muscle. And his lungs remained free of fluid during that time. The rabbi continued to require nutritional treatment for the rest of his life. However, these treatments allowed him to keep his legs and to maintain a reasonably healthy heart. He greatly outlived his doctors' expectations; the rabbi did not pass away after two weeks or a month, but rather, nearly eight years later, just before his eighty-seventh birthday.

Although results with nutritional therapy are not always as dramatic as this, it is common for individuals suffering from any of a wide range of conditions to find relief from *alternative* medicine, even after conventional methods have failed.

MEDICAL RESEARCH GATHERS DUST

From 1975 to the present, I have spent more than 10,000 hours spelunking the caves of medical libraries, where much wisdom and innovation lie gathering dust. This intensive search has turned up thousands of articles on nutritional therapy as it relates to the practice of medicine. Virtually none of this information was taught in medical school; nor could any of it be found in standard textbooks. However, since these treatments appeared to be safe, I tried them in my practice whenever appropriate. Most worked just as the articles said they would, but a few treatments did not and were abandoned.

As a result of this intensive review of the medical literature, combined with excellent training by my mentor, Jonathan V. Wright, M.D., of Kent, Washington, my patients frequently have better results, fewer side effects, and lower medical bills than their friends who seek conventional medical care. The nutritional approach, which makes use of dietary modifications and supplementation with vitamins, minerals, hormones, plant extracts, and other naturally occurring substances, is successful against a wide range of conditions, including fatigue, depression, heart disease, diabetes, high blood pressure, asthma, migraines, skin disorders, prostate enlargement, menstrual problems, recurrent infections, autoimmune disorders, gastrointestinal diseases, and arthritis. Recognizing the importance of this new approach to medicine, Dr. Wright and I have for the past ten years presented seminars on nutritional medicine to more than 2,000 health care practitioners. Currently, the Wright/Gaby research library contains more than 23,000 scientific papers related to nutritional and natural medicine.

LITTLE KNOWN RESEARCH ON OSTEOPOROSIS

While collecting articles over the years, I came across many that suggested there is more to osteoporosis treatment than calcium, estrogen, and exercise. During the past five years, the number of published articles supporting that point of view has increased dramatically. However, virtually none of this information has made it into standard textbooks or review articles on osteoporosis, and none of it was explored by the media. Interestingly, although many different investigators were reporting provocative findings, no one seemed to be communicating with their colleagues in a way that would help them recognize the patterns emerging from their research or the new concepts that followed logically from what they had discovered.

This inability to merge such data into a unifying thesis is unfortunately typical of scientists who do not believe that the degenerative diseases of modern civilization are caused in part by chronic nutritional deficiencies, hormonal imbalances, and environmental pollution. However, to this proponent of nutritional medicine, one who also believes that eclectic synthesis is not only a path to truth, but also an art, the research eventually reached a critical mass. Osteoporosis was looking more and more like other chronic diseases (such as heart disease, diabetes, asthma, and kidney stones), in that dietary modification, nutritional supplementation, hormone balancing, and avoidance of environmental toxins seemed to be more important than generally recognized. In the summer of 1992, I became convinced that there is an untold story about osteoporosis.

NEW CONCEPTS ABOUT OSTEOPOROSIS

Three major new concepts emerged from my review of the medical literature. First, is the idea that certain vitamins and minerals besides calcium play an important role in maintaining bone mass and preventing osteoporosis. Deficiencies of these nutrients are probably widespread among Americans, either because our typical processed diet is depleted of many vitamins and minerals, or because the massive pollution of our food, water, and air has increased our requirement for these nutrients. Whatever the reason, there is now evidence that supplementation with appropriate vitamins and minerals in addition to calcium is another key weapon in the battle against osteoporosis. In addition, certain aspects of our diet and lifestyle determine in part whether our bones will stand up to the demands of old age.

Second, estrogen is not the only hormone that has an important influence on the health of bones. Indeed, it may not even be the most significant hormone where osteoporosis is concerned. At least two other hormones produced by the ovaries, progesterone and dehydroepiandrosterone (DHEA), have a major influence on bone metabolism. Testosterone supplementation may also be of value in some cases. It is becoming increasingly clear that providing a proper balance of several hormones is more logical than using estrogen alone. An appropriate combination of hormones, possibly in lower doses, may not only be more effective against osteoporosis, but might also greatly reduce the risk of cancer associated with estrogen therapy.

Third, growing evidence suggests that pollution of our environment and contamination of our food—particularly with heavy metals such as aluminum, cadmium, lead, and tin—contributes to the development of osteoporosis. Other environmental chemicals, food additives, and even some prescription medications, may also play a role. Furthermore, acid rain has the capacity to cause bone loss in several different ways. The proliferation of environmental pollution and of acid rain during the past three decades coincides with the increasing incidence of osteoporosis in that time period.

WHERE'S THE PROOF?

It would be easy for skeptics to dismiss the evidence presented in this book as "unproven." As a scientist, I agree that some of what you are going to read is unproven. However, as a physician and a concerned citizen, I see this information as an opportunity for you to keep your bones strong and to enhance your general health. Opponents of the natural approach to medicine often forget that most of the treatments doctors prescribe every day are unproven. And some of those treatments are quite dangerous. The evidence supporting a new approach to the prevention and treatment of osteoporosis is at least as good as that supporting many conventional treatments.

Because of the heterogeneous nature of the human population, and because of the logistical and financial limitations that characterize medical research, physicians are often faced with making decisions on the basis of incomplete information. In other words, although doctors might not like to admit it, we make a lot of (hopefully educated) guesses. It is especially difficult to obtain proof of effectiveness where osteoporosis is concerned because it takes years for changes in bone mass and fracture incidence to become evident. Any definitive study of osteoporosis must therefore be continued over a long period of time. In addition, such studies are rather costly to perform because they involve state-of-the-art, expensive bone density measurements. When nonpatentable natural substances are involved, the roadblocks to performing convincing research become even more formidable. This is because most research grant money comes from the pharmaceutical industry and from other organizations that have a vested interest in studying patentable substances or in promoting a particular point of view.

If we spent even 10% of our research dollars investigating natural products, we would probably be much closer to solving the problem of osteoporosis. However, I believe the argument in favor of a new approach to osteoporosis is already quite compelling. Proving the case for this new approach will take time, partly because of the resistance of the medical establishment to new ideas, and partly because it takes years for changes in bone mass and fracture incidence to become measurable. Additional research also needs to be done so that we can "fine tune" our recommendations. However, on the basis of research that has already been published, I believe it is fair to conclude that there is, indeed, new hope for osteoporosis.

1

Overview of Osteoporosis

FACTORS RELATED TO FRACTURES

Osteoporosis is defined as thin or porous bones. Although bones generally become thinner in everyone with advancing age, some individuals develop osteoporosis so severe that their risk of breaking bones increases. Three major types of fractures result from osteoporosis. One is the spontaneous *vertebral crush fracture,* in which one of the vertebrae in the spine becomes so weak that it collapses under the minimal stress of lifting an object or even from the stress of the body's weight. Repeated vertebral crush fractures result in a loss of height. In addition, since most of these fractures occur on the anterior (front) side of the vertebra, repeated fractures cause the typical hunched over appearance characteristic of many elderly women. A second type of osteoporotic fracture, known as a *Colles' fracture,* occurs when a person lands on his or her hands while breaking a fall. Because the bones in the wrist and forearm have been weakened by osteoporosis, the trauma from the fall causes a fracture of the lower end of the radius (one of the two major bones in the forearm). The third and most serious type is the

1

osteoporotic hip fracture. As many as 20% of individuals who suffer a hip fracture die within one year, usually as a result of complications of the fracture. Up to 50% of elderly people end up in a nursing home after sustaining a hip fracture, and many others never recover the full function they had prior to the fracture. Although osteoporosis occurs in both sexes, the overwhelming majority of cases occur in women.

Thus, osteoporosis is a major cause of both morbidity and mortality, particularly among women. Nearly one-third of all American women will, during their lifetime, develop osteoporosis severe enough to cause a fracture. At least 1.2 million fractures (primarily of the types mentioned) occur each year in the United States as a direct result of osteoporosis. The medical and social costs of this epidemic are estimated to be $6.1 billion annually.[1]

In healthy individuals bones grow and develop during childhood and adolescence. Bones continue to become thicker and stronger during early adulthood, with peak bone mass occurring around age thirty-five in most women. Thereafter, bone mineral content begins to decline. This decline proceeds slowly in women until menopause, at which time bone loss accelerates rapidly for a period of eight to ten years. Thereafter, bone loss continues, but at a slower rate.

A NEW EPIDEMIC?

Although osteoporosis was recognized in antiquity, it was apparently not a common condition. As late as the nineteenth century, pathologists recognized fragile and osteoporotic bone not as a frequent occurrence, but as a medical curiosity.[2] Osteoporosis began to attract attention only after World War I. It has been suggested that this new interest in osteoporosis was due partly to the new availability of X rays and partly to increasing lifespans. However, those two factors could not be the entire explanation. Although the average lifespan may have been shorter in centuries past, some people still lived into their eighties and nineties. Furthermore, if osteoporosis were a common condition, pathologists should have been able to recognize it on routine autopsies. It is therefore likely that the increasing attention to osteoporosis in the early twentieth century was due, at least in part, to an increased prevalence of the condition.

The possibility that osteoporosis is largely a disease of modern civilization is supported by recent epidemiologic studies from Europe. In a survey of female residents of Nottingham, England, the annual incidence of hip fractures in those over the age of seventy-five increased from 8 per 1,000 in 1971 to 16 per 1,000 in 1981.[3] In another study of English citizens, the age-adjusted incidence of hip fractures nearly doubled between 1956 and 1983.[4] Similar findings have been reported from Sweden, where the incidence of hip fractures among individuals eighty years or older doubled between 1950 and 1981.[5] This rising incidence of osteoporotic fractures is not limited to the hip. In another study, the age-adjusted incidence of forearm fractures in residents of Malmö, Sweden, also doubled during the twenty-five-year period between 1955 and 1980.[6] Although data from the earlier part of this century are not available, these reports are consistent with the possibility that the prevalence of osteoporosis has been steadily increasing over the past one hundred years.

The recent restoration of a London church, during which skeletons dating from 1729 to 1852 were recovered, has provided scientists with an opportunity to compare the rate of bone loss then and now. The rate of bone loss in the hip was found to be significantly greater in modern-day women than in the women from two centuries ago, both before and after menopause.[7] These findings indicate that osteoporosis is more common today than it was in the past.

The possible relationship between modern civilization and osteoporosis is further supported by investigations of individuals in developing countries. In Surinam, South America, for example, the prevalence and severity of osteoporosis among individuals ages 67 to 94 was considerably less than that reported for elderly Americans, even though the average daily calcium intake in Surinam is less than that consumed by the typical American.[8] Similar findings have been reported for people living in other developing nations. If osteoporosis is, indeed, more prevalent in modern societies, then the causes of this condition are probably related in part to changes in our diet and our environment. This book identifies a number of nutritional and environmental factors that might be related to this apparently new epidemic.

OTHER CAUSES OF OSTEOPOROSIS

Osteoporosis can occur in association with a number of endocrine conditions, including diabetes, thyrotoxicosis (overactive thyroid gland), Cushing's syndrome (excessive secretion of adrenal hormones), and hyperparathyroidism (excessive secretion of parathyroid hormone). Rheumatoid arthritis and chronic lung disease are also associated with an increased risk of osteoporosis. Certain prescription drugs may increase the likelihood of developing bone loss. These include adrenal corticosteroids (cortisonelike drugs), anticonvulsants, anticoagulants, aluminum-containing antacids, some cancer chemotherapy medications, phenothiazine derivatives, lithium, tetracycline, and loop diuretics (such as furosemide).[9] In addition, both excessive alcohol intake and cigarette smoking have been reported to promote osteoporosis.

BONES ARE LIVING TISSUE

We sometimes forget that bone is more than just a collection of calcium crystals. Bone is active, living tissue, continually remodeling itself and constantly participating in a wide range of biochemical reactions. Bone tissue consists of both cells and an intercellular matrix. *Osteoblasts* are the cells within bone involved in laying down new bone tissue. *Osteoclasts*, on the other hand, participate in the breaking down of old or damaged bone tissue (a process called **resorption**). The formation and resorption of bone are dynamic processes, which occur in all bones throughout life. This process of resorption coupled with new bone formation is called **remodeling**.

Bone remodeling serves two purposes. First, it helps keep bones "young," by replacing old or weakened areas with new, well-formed tissue. If, for example, a repetitive, stressful activity produces microscopic areas of fatigue-fracture in a bone, that bone will be more susceptible to breaking. By replacing the fatigue-fractured area with new bone, the bone becomes reinforced and more resistant to stress. The second function of bone remodeling is to make the bone better able to meet the everyday demands that are placed on it. For example, in tennis players the humerus (the large bone in the upper arm) in the playing arm usually becomes thicker and stronger than that in the other arm. Thus, bone remodels itself along the lines of repetitive stress, thereby increasing its ability to deal with that stress.

The intercellular matrix of bone consists of an organic component, primarily collagen and other proteins, and an inorganic component, which is responsible for the rigidity of bone. The inorganic component is composed mainly of calcium phosphate and calcium carbonate, with small amounts of magnesium, fluoride, sulfate, and other trace minerals. These minerals form crystals known as *hydroxyapatites*.

While the risk of developing fractures is definitely related to bone mass (that is, bone mineral content), thinning of the bones may not by itself be sufficient to result in a fracture. Why is it that some individuals with a given bone mineral content suffer repeated fractures, while others with the same bone mass do just fine? Several other factors that influence the strength and resistance of bone tissue, independent of its mineral content, have been identified. One factor is the integrity of the protein matrix and the other supporting structures in bone. A second factor is the efficiency with which the bone can repair the accumulation of microfractures resulting from repeated mild trauma. Thus, the overall structure and function of bone tissue is important, not just the absolute amount of inorganic mineral present. Preventing fractures therefore requires attention to at least three factors: (1) preventing loss of calcium and other minerals from bone, (2) maintaining the soft tissue components of bone, such as proteins, which give bones their unique structure, and (3) making sure that bones are capable of efficiently repairing damaged areas.

A COMPREHENSIVE APPROACH

While there is no proven method guaranteed to achieve all of these objectives, careful attention to nutritional and hormonal factors is no doubt important. Like other tissues in the body, bone is complex, living tissue with diverse nutritional and hormonal needs. Failure to meet any one of these needs could presumably compromise the strength and integrity of bone tissue. Bones are made up of much more than just calcium. As future chapters will show, magnesium is necessary to promote normal bone mineralization; silicon, manganese, and vitamin C are essential for proper formation of cartilage and other organic components of bone; vitamin K is needed to attract calcium to the bones; vitamin D is necessary for absorption of calcium from the diet; and zinc and copper are involved in repair mechanisms, presumably including those that occur in bone. Estrogen has been shown to inhibit bone resorption, while progesterone and possibly dehydroepiandrosterone (DHEA) promote bone formation.

As you can see, a lot of complicated events are occurring in bone tissue every minute of every day. We still do not have a complete understanding of how all of the nutrients and hormones interact. However, there is enough evidence now for us to make interim recommendations about nutritional supplementation and hormonal therapy. That is what this book is about.

The typical Western diet, with its high proportion of refined sugar, white flour, fat, and canned foods, contains far less of certain vitamins and minerals than diets consumed by our ancestors. Furthermore, the requirement for certain nutrients may be increased by genetic factors, environmental pollution, or metabolic changes that occur around the time of menopause. Inadequate intake of any one of these nutrients could play a role in the development of osteoporosis. Multiple deficiencies over a prolonged period of time may have even greater significance. This possibility is supported by the work of Dr. Anthony A. Albanese, who found that adding "all known micronutrients" to a calcium supplement reduced bone loss to a significantly greater degree than calcium alone.[10] Some of the nutrients that play a role in maintaining healthy bones are discussed later in this book.

Other potentially important factors that will be discussed are the role of diet and lifestyle; hormonal replacement therapy (including certain lesser known hormones); exercise; and avoidance of environmental pollutants. When scientists study the "diseases of modern civilization," they usually find that many different factors contribute to the cause of the disease. For example, heart disease seems to be caused in part by excessive dietary fat and sugar, lack of exercise, and deficiencies of vitamin C, vitamin E, beta-carotene, vitamin B6, chromium, magnesium, and other nutrients. It is likely that, when all of the information is in on osteoporosis, it, too, will be known as a multifactorial disease. That is why it is best to look for and correct as many contributing factors as possible.

NOTES

1. Riggs, B. L., and L. J. Melton III. 1986. Involutional osteoporosis. *N Engl J Med* 314:1676–1686.
2. Frost, H. M. 1985. The pathomechanics of osteoporoses. *Clin Orthop* 200:198–225.
3. Wallace, W. A. 1983. The increasing incidence of fractures of the proximal femur: An orthopaedic epidemic. *Lancet* 1:1413–1414.
4. Boyce, W. J., and M. P. Vessey. 1985. Rising incidence of fracture of the proximal femur. *Lancet* 1:150–151.
5. Johnell, O., et al. 1984. Age and sex patterns of hip fracture—changes in 30 years. *Acta Orthop Scand* 55:290–292.
6. Bengner, U., and O. Johnell. 1985. Increasing incidence of forearm fractures. A comparison of epidemiologic patterns 25 years apart. *Acta Orthop Scand* 56:158–160.
7. Lees, B., et al. 1993. Differences in proximal femur bone density over two centuries. *Lancet* 341:673–675.
8. Zeegelaar, F. J., et al. 1967. Studies on physiology of nutrition in Surinam. XI. The skeleton of aged people in Surinam. *Am J Clin Nutr* 20:43–45.
9. Avioli, L. V. 1990. Therapy induced osteoporosis (??? Type III osteoporosis). In *Osteoporosis: Physiological basis, assessment, and treatment,* edited by H. F. Deluca and R. Mazess, 17. New York: Elsevier.
10. Albanese, A. A., et al. 1981. Effects of calcium and micronutrients on bone loss of pre- and postmenopausal women. Scientific exhibit presented to the American Medical Association, 24–26 January, in Atlanta, Georgia.

2

What You Eat Affects Your Bones

THE HIPPOCRATIC OATH

In the practice of medicine one basic principle stands out: What you eat has a major influence on your health. That principle is so simple and so logical that it is surprising the medical profession has had such a difficult time grasping it. The average doctor, despite having taken the Hippocratic oath, rejects the famous words proclaimed by Hippocrates: "Let your food be your medicine and let your medicine be your food." Had these doctors only met my late Uncle Ruben, who, well into his nineties, was still able to walk a brisk five miles every morning, they would have understood why he believed that "health comes from the farm, not the pharmacy."

A theme that keeps recurring in nutritional medicine is that degenerative diseases are caused, at least in part, by our modern diet, which contains too much sugar, fat, salt, refined flour, caffeine, alcohol, processed foods, and food additives. I routinely advise my patients, regardless of their specific medical problems, to try to "clean up" their diet; that is, reduce their consumption of these "junk foods" and to increase their intake of whole grains, fruits, vegetables, nuts and seeds, beans, and other unprocessed foods. The majority of people who follow that advice find that their health improves in some way. Many individuals report an increase in energy, less depression and anxiety, fewer headaches, better bowel and bladder function, and less fluid retention. They often sleep better, their joints do not hurt as much, and they are more alert and productive. Laboratory reports, such as serum cholesterol, triglycerides, liver enzymes, and uric acid also improve in many cases.

Specific medical conditions may also be relieved as a result of these general dietary changes. Patients with asthma, irritable bowel syndrome, peptic ulcer, gallbladder attacks, acne, psoriasis, high blood pressure, diabetes, angina, or other problems frequently find that their symptoms are better when they eat a healthier diet. Part of the appeal of improving your diet is that, even if it does not help, it rarely causes harm.

DIET AND BONE HEALTH

Considering that bone is living tissue, just like the rest of the body, it is likely that what you put in your mouth will determine in part how strong your bones will be. Many people believe that, aside from its calcium content, diet has little to do with osteoporosis. However, that assumption ignores the fact that bone tissue has diverse nutritional needs and engages in complex interactions with the rest of the body. It is improbable that our modern-day diet could be sparing our bones while damaging the rest of our body. Although it is impossible to determine the precise effect of diet on bone health, there is at least circumstantial evidence that the typical American diet promotes the development of osteoporosis.

There are three reasons that our modern diet might not be good for our bones. First, many of us ingest too much sugar, caffeine, salt, and alcohol. Consumption of each of these substances is reportedly associated with an increased risk of osteoporosis. Second, because of the way our food is grown and refined, today's diet probably contains much lower quantities of various vitamins and minerals than it used to. As you will learn later, some of these vitamins and minerals play a key role in maintaining healthy bones. Third, some of the processing techniques used by the food industry cause chemical changes in our food that may adversely affect the health of the tissues in our bodies, including bone. The possible influences of diet on bone health are reviewed next.

Sugar

In the early part of the nineteenth century, sugar was considered a condiment, rather than a major component of the diet. Back then, the average per capita intake of sugar was only about 10 to 12 pounds per year. Today, according to some statistics, the average American ingests approximately 139 pounds of refined sugar each year. That enormous quantity translates to about 41 teaspoons of sugar per day, or 19% of all of the calories we consume. Since refined sugar contains virtually no vitamins or minerals at all, it dilutes our nutrient intake, resulting in an across-the-board 19% reduction in all vitamins and minerals in our diet. Thus, because of our high intake of sugar we are getting less magnesium, folic acid, vitamin B6, zinc, copper, manganese, and other nutrients that play a role in maintaining healthy bones.

Ingesting sugar may also deplete our bodies of calcium. In one study, administering 100 grams (about 25 teaspoons) of sugar (sucrose) to healthy volunteers caused a significant increase in the urinary excretion of calcium. When the same amount of sugar was given to people with a history of calcium oxalate kidney stones or to their relatives, the increase in calcium excretion was even greater.[1] Since 99% of the total-body calcium is in our bones, this increase in calcium excretion most likely reflects a leaching of calcium from bone. This study suggests that a high-sugar diet may reduce the calcium content of bone, and that people with kidney stones or their relatives are especially susceptible to the adverse effects of sugar. Thus, the extent to which dietary sugar affects calcium metabolism is in part genetically determined, just as there is a hereditary component to osteoporosis risk. It is interesting to note that individuals with a history of kidney stones are at increased risk for developing osteoporosis.[2] Researchers have also suggested that consumption of refined sugar is one of the factors that promotes kidney stones. Perhaps what people with kidney stones and osteoporosis have in common is an increased sensitivity to refined sugar.

Ingestion of large amounts of sugar has another effect on the body that may promote osteoporosis. Dr. John Yudkin, a British physician, has been studying the effects of dietary sugar for more than thirty years. Yudkin found that ingesting large amounts of sucrose by healthy volunteers causes a significant increase in the fasting serum cortisol level. Cortisol is the primary corticosteroid (cortisonelike hormone) secreted by the adrenal gland. Although corticosteroids have important biological functions, an excess of these hormones can cause osteoporosis. Indeed, doctors are reluctant to prescribe corticosteroids precisely because they can cause severe bone loss. Yudkin's work demonstrated that eating too much sugar is in a way analogous to taking a small amount of cortisone, which could cause your bones to become thinner. This possibility is supported by a study on hamsters, in which feeding a diet containing 56% sucrose caused osteoporosis, despite adequate intake of calcium.[3]

Refined Grains and Flour

Another significant dietary change occurring during the past century is an increase in the consumption of refined grains, such as white bread instead of whole wheat bread, and white rice instead of brown rice. During the refining of grains and flour the nutrient-rich germ and bran portions are removed, resulting in a significant loss of vitamins and minerals. For example, when whole wheat is refined to white flour the following percentages of selected vitamins and minerals are lost: vitamin B6 (72%), folic acid (67%), calcium (60%), magnesium (85%), manganese (86%), copper (68%), zinc (78%).[4] Since grains make up about 30% of the average diet, consumption of refined grains would have a substantial impact on the total daily intake of micronutrients (vitamins and minerals). Because nearly 50% of the typical American diet is composed of nutrient-depleted sugar and refined grains, the intake of many important micronutrients is probably much lower than it was during the previous century.

Caffeine

Caffeine is found in coffee, tea, cola beverages, and certain pain medications. Substances similar to caffeine are also present in chocolate. Caffeine has certain pharmacologic (druglike) effects in the human body and is known primarily as a stimulant of the central nervous system. Tens of millions of people depend on caffeine to help them wake up in the morning and to stay alert during the day. Athletes sometimes use caffeine to enhance their performance.

Although the dangers of caffeine have long been a topic of debate, it is well known that caffeine is an addictive substance. Withdrawal from caffeine after prolonged use usually results in severe headaches, which can last several days. It is also well known that excessive caffeine use is a cause of anxiety and insomnia.

Nutrition-oriented practitioners and some conventional doctors believe that caffeine can also cause certain other problems in susceptible individuals. Problems attributed wholly or in part to caffeine include fibrocystic breast disease, cardiac arrhythmias (heart rhythm disturbances), diarrhea, constipation, abdominal pain, elevated serum cholesterol or blood sugar, high blood pressure, and chronic migraines or other headaches. There is evidence that caffeine may also promote heart disease and cancer, although the studies in this area are conflicting.

It should not be surprising that a substance that appears to cause problems in so many different systems of the body would also adversely affect bone tissue. Most of the evidence is circumstantial, but studies do suggest that caffeine ingestion may contribute to bone loss. In one study, thirty-one women ingested a cup of decaffeinated coffee on three different occasions. In two of the cups, caffeine was added at concentrations of 3 mg/kg and 6 mg/kg of body weight, respectively. The excretion of calcium in the urine during the next three hours was signficantly greater after caffeine ingestion than after decaffeinated coffee. The increases in calcium excretion were 50% and 69%, respectively, after low and high doses of caffeine.[5] These results demonstrate that ingestion of caffeine causes excess calcium loss from the body in the short term.

Another study suggests that this effect of caffeine is not just limited to the short term. Calcium balance, a measure of the amount of calcium retained in the body, was assessed in 168 women between the ages of 35 and 45. The results showed that calcium balance decreased with increasing dietary intake of caffeine. In other words, women who habitually ingested a great deal of caffeine retained less calcium than did those who used little caffeine. Women who consumed 50% more caffeine than average had an estimated reduction in calcium balance of 6 mg/day.[6] Although 6 mg/day might seem like a small amount, a loss of that much calcium every day for years would add up to a significant degree of bone loss.

The potential consequences of caffeine ingestion on bone health was assessed in a study of 84,484 women between the ages of 34 and 59. In 1980, each of the women completed a questionnaire pertaining to their intake of various foods and beverages. During the ensuing six years, there was a positive association between caffeine intake and the risk of sustaining a hip fracture. That is, the risk of a hip fracture increased with increasing levels of caffeine intake. Women who consumed the most caffeine (above the 80th percentile) had nearly three times as many hip fractures as women who consumed the least caffeine (below the 20th percentile).[7] One possible confounding factor in this study is that women who use caffeine also tend to smoke cigarettes, which are known to contribute to the risk of osteoporosis. It is possible that some of the risk attributed to caffeine intake was actually due to tobacco. However, the weight of evidence suggests that anyone interested in maintaining healthy bones should avoid excessive caffeine intake.

Alcohol

Consumption of excessive amounts of alcohol is a known risk factor for osteoporosis. In a study of ninety-six male chronic alcoholics, ages 24 to 62, 47% had osteoporosis. Among those under the age of 40, 31% had osteoporosis.[8] Although a similar study has not been done on women, it is likely that drinking too much alcohol would also promote osteoporosis in women. The effect of moderate alcohol consumption on bone health is not known.

Protein, Phosphorus, and Sodium

The American diet tends to contain too much, rather than too little protein. Studies have shown that excessive dietary protein may promote bone loss. With increasing protein intake, the urinary excretion of calcium also rises, because calcium is mobilized to buffer the acidic breakdown products of protein. In addition, the amino acid methionine is converted to a substance called homocysteine, which is also apparently capable of causing bone loss.

Animal studies have shown that excessive intake of phosphorus can cause oteoporosis, as well. The effect of dietary protein on osteoporosis might be explained in part by the phosphorus content of many high-protein foods because phosphorus does appear to have an adverse effect on bone health. High-phosphorus beverages such as colas (which also contain a lot of sugar and caffeine) are among the worst foods imaginable for someone trying to prevent osteoporosis.

Several studies have shown that individuals who consume a vegetarian diet have stronger bones later in life than those who eat animal flesh.[9,10] However, other studies have failed to find a difference in bone mass between vegetarians and meat eaters.

A substantial minority of human beings also appears to be susceptible to the effects of high-sodium intake. When these individuals ingest moderate amounts of salt, their urinary excretion of calcium increases markedly.[11] In people with this "sodium-dependent hypercalciuria," ingestion of too much salt probably increases the risk of both kidney stones and osteoporosis.

Food Processing

In today's fast paced society, great emphasis is placed on readily available, easily prepared food, which can be stored on the shelf for prolonged periods of time. The food technology industry has developed many ways to achieve these goals. Unfortunately, the nutritional quality of processed, adulterated food is far inferior to that of fresh, perishable foods. Modern food is bleached, radiated, extracted with organic solvents, subjected to enormous temperatures and extremes of acidity or alkalinity, and contaminated with thousands of chemicals designed to preserve, texturize, color, or otherwise modify the food so that it will look, feel, and taste like the real thing.

Hundreds of articles have been written about how these harsh processing techniques can affect the nutritional value of food. One example is the possibility that food processing can promote lysine deficiency. Lysine is one of the eight essential amino acids from which protein molecules are synthesized in the body. Studies have shown that when proteins are subjected to alkali treatment (as in the production of isolated soy protein or textured vegetable protein), a substantial amount of the lysine is destroyed.[12] Exposure of lysine to temperatures of 250°C for one hour also caused significant losses of lysine.[13] Heating proteins even at moderate temperatures in the presence of sugars such as lactose, glucose, or sucrose can also destroy significant amounts of lysine.[14] Thus, in the baking of pies, cookies, breads, and other grain products, where flour and sugar are heated together, substantial amounts of lysine may be lost.

You might assume that, with all of the protein in the American diet, it would be difficult to develop a *deficiency* of an amino acid. The problem is, however, that amino acid *imbalance* can be just as damaging as amino acid deficiency. Animal studies have shown that the *ratios* of essential amino acids in the diet are as important as the *absolute* amount of each. If a single amino acid, such as lysine, is being systematically destroyed by food processing, then ingesting more of all of the amino acids will not correct a relative lack of lysine.

It is therefore possible that millions of Americans are marginally deficient in lysine, even if their diet is high in protein. The modern epidemic of herpes simplex infections is certainly consistent with that possibility. Lysine is known to inhibit the growth of herpes viruses and oral supplementation with lysine has been shown to prevent recurrences of herpes simplex outbreaks in susceptible individuals.[15,16] Since the doses of lysine that were effective against herpes infections (312 to 3,000 mg/day) are similar to the amounts obtainable in the diet, it is possible that dietary lysine deficiency is a factor in the increased incidence of herpes simplex infections.

It is also possible that lysine deficiency contributes to the development of osteoporosis. Individuals with a rare genetic condition known as lysinuric protein intolerance develop osteoporosis during childhood. In lysinuric protein intolerance, a defect in the kidneys causes large amounts of lysine to be lost in the urine. Scientists have suggested that lysine deficiency is the cause of osteoporosis in individuals with this disorder.[17] Although the typical American diet would not result in lysine deficiency that severe, it is possible that prolonged, subtle lysine deficiency caused by harsh food processing techniques could have an adverse effect on bones.

Soil Factors

The reduction in vitamin and mineral intake resulting from refining of foods can be made even worse by farming techniques that deplete the soil of essential minerals. Traditional methods of farming include using manure and compost to increase the trace mineral content of the soil. In modern times, however, with the emphasis on producing higher crop yields per acre, farmers use large amounts of inorganic fertilizers, which are often deficient in important trace minerals and which may disturb soil mineral balance. For example, the use of ammonia as a fertilizer causes essential minerals such as magnesium, manganese, zinc, and copper to be leached from the soil.[18] Repeated application of inorganic fertilizers, which are low in essential trace minerals, can further reduce the soil concentration of these trace minerals.

Many scientists and nutritionists are unaware of the effect that depleted soil can have on the mineral content of edible plants. Indeed, nutrition textbooks often contend that mineral-deficient soil will reduce crop yield, but will not adversely affect the nutritional quality of crops that do grow. However, the facts indicate otherwise. The presence of a "goiter belt" in the midwestern United States attests to the fact that foods grown on iodine-deficient soil can cause iodine deficiency. The relationship between mineral concentrations in soil and food is also underscored by the epidemics of selenium deficiency that have occurred in cattle grazing in low-selenium areas of the country. As another example, dairy cattle and horses are sometimes stricken by a condition known as grass staggers, characterized by unsteady gait and twitching and spasm of the muscles. This disorder can be cured either by supplementing the diet with magnesium or by adding magnesium to the soil.[19] It appears that overuse of nitrates, phosphates, and potassium salts as fertilizers depletes the soil of magnesium and causes a deficiency of this mineral in grazing animals. In the Florida Everglades the soil is low in copper. Domestic animals grazing in this area develop copper deficiency which makes them unusually susceptible to sustaining bone fractures. But, when copper is added to their diet fractures no longer occur.[20] In another study, the manganese content of turnips was directly related to the manganese content of the soil. Addition of calcium carbonate to the soil (a common practice by modern farmers) decreased the accumulation of manganese by turnips.[21]

CONCLUSION

These studies indicate that modern farming practices deplete the soil of essential minerals, resulting in lower levels of these minerals in our food. The vitamin and mineral content of our diet is further reduced by overconsumption of nutrient-depleted foods, such as sugar and white flour. The net result is that the food we consume today contains far less of many vitamins and minerals than it did in the past. One of the major theses of this book is that chronic, low-level deficiencies of a wide range of micronutrients may increase the risk of developing osteoporosis.

In summary, many factors related to the modern American diet may promote not only osteoporosis, but other chronic diseases, as well. A health-promoting diet is one that emphasizes fresh, unprocessed foods, such as whole grains, fruits and vegetables, nuts and seeds, and legumes. Animal foods, dairy products, and salt should be used in moderation, and sweets, caffeine, refined flours, and chemical food additives should be avoided as much as possible. While some studies suggest that moderate alcohol intake improves health, others have shown that even small amounts of alcohol are not good for you. Certainly, excessive alcohol intake can cause many different problems, including osteoporosis. The human body is remarkably resilient and is capable of withstanding numerous stresses, but it is also true that the more closely you follow the principles of good eating, the healthier you will be.

NOTES

1. Lemann, J., Jr., W. F. Piering, and E. J. Lennon. 1969. Possible role of carbohydrate-induced calciuria in calcium oxalate kidney-stone formation. *N Engl J Med* 280:232–237.
2. Lawoyin, S., et al. 1979. Bone mineral content in patients with calcium urolithiasis. *Metabolism* 28:1250–1254.
3. Yudkin, J., Dr. 1973. *Sweet and dangerous.* New York: Bantam Books, 112. Saffar, J. L., et al. 1981. Osteoporotic effect of a high-carbohydrate diet (Keyes 2000) in golden hamsters. *Arch Oral Biol* 26:393–397.
4. Schroeder, H. A. 1971. Losses of vitamins and trace minerals resulting from processing and preservation of foods. *Am J Clin Nutr* 24:562–573.
5. Hollingbery, P. W., E. A. Bergman, and L. K. Massey. 1985. Effect of dietary caffeine and aspirin on urinary calcium and hydroxyproline excretion in pre- and postmenopausal women. *Fed Proc* 44:1149.
6. Heaney, R. P., and R. R. Recker. 1982. Effects of nitrogen, phosphorus, and caffeine on calcium balance in women. *J Lab Clin Med* 99:46–55.
7. Hernandez-Avila, M., et al. 1991. Caffeine, moderate alcohol intake, and risk of fractures of the hip and forearm in middle-aged women. *Am J Clin Nutr* 54:157–163.
8. Spencer, H., et al. 1985. Alcohol-osteoporosis. *Am J Clin Nutr* 41:847.

9. Marsh, A. G., et al. 1980. Cortical bone density of adult lacto-ovo-vegetarian and omnivorous women. *J Am Diet Assoc* 76:148–151.

10. Marsh, A. G., et al. 1983. Bone mineral mass in adult lacto-ovo-vegetarian and omnivorous males. *Am J Clin Nutr* 37:453–456.

11. Silver, J., et al. 1983. Sodium-dependent idiopathic hypercalciuria in renal-stone formers. *Lancet* 2:484–486.

12. de Groot, A. P., and P. Slump. 1969. Effects of severe alkali treatment of proteins on amino acid composition and nutritive value. *J Nutr* 98:45–56.

13. Breitbart, D. J., and W. W. Nawar. 1979. Thermal decomposition of lysine. *J Agric Food Chem* 27:511–514.

14. Hurrell, R. F., and K. J. Carpenter. 1977. Mechanisms of heat damage in proteins. 8. The role of sucrose in the susceptibility of protein foods to heat damage. *Br J Nutr* 38:285–297.

15. Griffith, R. S., A. L. Norins, and C. Kagan. 1978. A multicentered study of lysine therapy in herpes simplex infection. *Dermatologica* 156:257–267.

16. Griffith, R. S., et al. 1987. Success of L-lysine therapy in frequently recurrent herpes simplex infection. *Dermatologica* 175:183–190.

17. Carpenter, T. O., et al. 1985. Lysinuric protein intolerance presenting as childhood osteoporosis. *N Engl J Med* 312:290–294.

18. Hall, R. H. 1981. The agri-business view of soil and life. *J Holistic Med* 3:157–166.

19. Ebeling, W. 1981. The relation of soil quality to the nutritional value of plant crops. *J Appl Nutr* 33(1):19–34.

20. Rose, E. F. 1968. The effects of soil and diet on disease. *Cancer Res* 28:2390–2392.

21. Hopkins, H. T., E. H. Stevenson, and P. L. Harris. 1966. Soil factors and food composition. *Am J Clin Nutr* 18:390–395.

3

Vitamin K: As Important for Your Bones as Calcium

Vitamin K is often referred to as the clotting vitamin. It was assigned the letter *K* because of its ability to promote blood *Koagulation*. When the body sustains a cut or wound, certain proteins circulating in the bloodstream migrate to the bleeding site. Vitamin K converts these proteins into so-called clotting factors, which initiate the process of clotting and healing. Individuals who are deficient in vitamin K tend to bleed or bruise excessively.

Although biochemists have long been fascinated by the elegant and intricate role played by vitamin K in the clotting mechanism, nutritionists were, until recently, not very interested in this vitamin. After all, there was little you could do with vitamin K. Most people have normal blood clotting function, and in those who do not, vitamin K deficiency is hardly ever the cause of the problem. Furthermore, conventional wisdom holds that it is very difficult to become deficient in vitamin K. Since this vitamin is present in a wide variety of plant foods, particularly leafy green vegetables, every reasonably healthy diet contains at least some vitamin K. More important, some of the bacteria that normally reside in your intestinal tract manufacture significant amounts of vitamin K. Therefore, even if you hate vegetables, your intestinal flora will probably give you enough vitamin K to prevent bleeding problems.

VITAMIN K AND CALCIUM METABOLISM

New research on vitamin K has caused the medical community to rethink its nonchalant attitude toward this vitamin. It is now well documented that the role of vitamin K is not limited to blood clotting; it is also critically involved in maintaining healthy bones and preventing osteoporosis. Furthermore, with improvements in laboratory methods for measuring vitamin K status, it has become clear that subtle vitamin K deficiency may be much more common than anyone had previously thought. A strong case can now be made that vitamin K deficiency is one of the factors contributing to the development of osteoporosis, and that vitamin K supplementation may be of value in preventing or reversing bone loss.

Those of you who have never been exposed to the joys of learning biochemical pathways may wish merely to accept that vitamin K is involved in bone formation and skip the next two paragraphs. But if you're interested in the details, read on. Vitamin K is required for the production of *osteocalcin*, a protein found in large amounts in bone.[1] Osteocalcin was so named because it is found solely in bone ("osteo") and because it has certain chemical characteristics that cause it to attract calcium ("calcin") to bone tissue, enabling calcium crystal formation to occur. Osteocalcin is the protein matrix upon which mineralization occurs; it provides structure and order to bone tissue.

Normally, protein molecules do not attract calcium ions because proteins do not contain two adjacent negative charges necessary to attract the double-positive charges of calcium ions. However, vitamin K is capable of changing that. Vitamin K catalyzes a structural change in glutamic acid, one of the amino acid components of osteocalcin. In a process called gamma-carboxylation, vitamin K converts glutamic acid to gamma-carboxyglutamic acid (GIA). While glutamic acid contains only one negative charge, GIA has two adjacent negative charges, which attract calcium ions. The migration of calcium to the site of GLA molecules is a crucial step in the mineralization of bone. Thus, vitamin K plays a key role in the formation, remodeling, and repair of bone, by helping to build the protein matrix upon which calcium crystallizes. Without adequate vitamin K, bones would lack structure and order and would, like chalk, be fragile and easily broken.

DEFICIENCY MORE COMMON THAN BELIEVED

Although the role of vitamin K in bone metabolism has now been clearly documented, virtually no one in the medical community has considered the possibility that increasing one's vitamin K intake might help combat osteoporosis. That is because doctors have been taught that vitamin K deficiency is extremely rare and that supplementation is therefore unnecessary. Since individuals with osteoporosis are not typically troubled by abnormal bleeding, physicians have had no apparent reason to suspect that osteoporosis might be associated with vitamin K deficiency. In fact, measurements of prothrombin time, a standard blood clotting test which indirectly measures vitamin K status, suggest that vitamin K deficiency is extremely uncommon, regardless of whether or not someone has osteoporosis. Consequently, the newly discovered function of vitamin K in relation to bone mineralization was considered interesting, but not relevant to osteoporosis.

However, doctors failed to consider the possibility that prothrombin time is a relatively insensitive test that might fail to detect subtle deficiencies of vitamin K. Recent technical advances have made it possible for the first time to measure reliably vitamin K levels in the blood and to compare these levels in individuals with and without osteoporosis. Dr. J. P. Hart and associates from the Kennedy Institute of Rheumatology, London, England, measured serum vitamin K levels in sixteen patients with osteoporosis who had suffered a hip fracture within the previous forty-eight hours. Compared with a control group of fifteen apparently healthy individuals, the people with osteoporosis had on average 74% less vitamin K.[2] Although the fracture patients were somewhat older than the healthy controls (average age, 77 versus 63 years), a 74% decline seems too large to be explained by differences in age alone. A more likely explanation is that the acute stress caused by the hip fracture may have caused a short-term reduction in vitamin K levels. Perhaps some of the vitamin K was being mobilized from the serum to the fracture site, where it would promote fracture healing by aiding in the production of new bone tissue.

To address that possibility, Hart and associates also measured serum vitamin K levels in fourteen other individuals with osteoporosis who had experienced a spinal (vertebral) crush fracture between eight months and five years previously. The average age of these patients was seventy years, more similar to that of the control group. More important, since the spinal fractures were all old, any reduction in vitamin K levels due to the fracture itself would have long since been corrected. However, even in this group, there was a statistically significant 56% reduction in average serum vitamin K levels. These results indicate that fractures reduce serum vitamin K levels in the short term, but that osteoporosis per se is also associated with a substantial decline in serum vitamin K.

VITAMIN K AND OSTEOPOROSIS

Is the reduction in vitamin K levels found by Hart a cause or an effect of osteoporosis, or both? Or is it merely an incidental association that has no real significance? These questions cannot be answered with certainty. It is, of course, possible that vitamin K migrates from serum to bone in an attempt to rebuild osteoporotic bone. If that is the case, then the low serum vitamin K levels are a reflection of bone loss, rather than a cause.

On the other hand, there is reason to believe that low levels of vitamin K also contribute to the development of osteoporosis. In one study, rats made deficient in vitamin K by a combination of antibiotic treatment and a vitamin K–deficient diet had increased urinary excretion of calcium which returned to normal when vitamin K was restored to the diet.[3] Since vitamin K deficiency did not affect intestinal absorption of calcium, the increase in urinary calcium excretion was due to leaching of calcium from bone.

Research done with humans also suggests that the low levels of vitamin K seen in osteoporosis are clinically significant. In a study performed in Japan more than twenty years ago, administering vitamin K to three women with osteoporosis reduced calcium loss in the urine by 18 to 50%.[4] This study suggests that supplementing with vitamin K reduced the amount of calcium lost from the bones. These findings were confirmed and extended in a more recent study done at the University of Limburg in the Netherlands.[5] Researchers measured the capacity of osteocalcin (a bone protein) to bind hydroxyapatite (a type of calcium crystal found in bone). This test is an indirect measurement of how efficiently bone tissue can attract calcium to participate in mineralization. Among a group of fifty healthy postmenopausal women (aged 55 to 75), the capacity of osteocalcin to attract calcium was reduced by an average of more than 50%. However, after the women were given 1 mg/day of vitamin K for two weeks, the test became normal.

The results of this study suggest that postmenopausal women are not getting as much vitamin K as they need for optimal bone health. It seems likely that postmenopausal women need more vitamin K for bone health than they do for normal blood clotting. The Dutch researchers also found that nearly one-fourth of postmenopausal women have elevated urinary calcium excretion, probably because they are losing bone at an accelerated rate. In this group of "fast losers," administering vitamin K reduced calcium excretion by 33%, suggesting that bone loss had been slowed or stopped.[6]

Another important finding from the Dutch study is that most premenopausal women probably have adequate levels of vitamin K, whereas a significant proportion of postmenopausal women need more vitamin K than they are getting. There are two possible explanations for the relative lack of vitamin K in the older group of women. First, aging is often accompanied by reduced intake of food, particularly fresh green vegetables, and by less-efficient nutrient absorption across the gastrointestinal tract. As a result, postmenopausal women may be getting less vitamin K into their bodies than they used to. Second, changes in hormone and bone metabolism

associated with menopause may somehow increase the requirement for vitamin K. Whatever the explanation, the evidence suggests
that postmenopausal women, ~~particularly those with accelerated
bone loss and/or osteoporosis, can benefit by increasing their intake of vitamin K.~~

VITAMIN K AND FRACTURES

A study on the role of vitamin K in fracture healing provides additional support for the concept that this vitamin promotes healthy
bones. In an experiment performed in Belgium in 1960, rabbits and
rats receiving well-balanced diets were subjected to fractures of the
tibia, a large bone in the lower leg. Even though their diet contained
adequate amounts of all known nutrients, the animals given additional vitamin K healed faster than the others.[7] Fracture healing
involves rapid production of new bone. Likewise, prevention and
reversal of osteoporosis requires efficient formation of new bone.
To the extent that vitamin K enhances bone formation, it would be
of value in both fracture healing and osteoporosis.

Studies by Hart and associates also provide evidence that vitamin K is important for healing fractures.[8] These researchers found
that, when nonosteoporotic individuals break a bone, serum vitamin
K levels fall by as much as 71%, and that these levels remain low
as long as fracture healing is taking place. This study suggests that
vitamin K migrates from the blood to the fracture site where it
participates in the healing process.

WHY VITAMIN K DEFICIENCY?

If vitamin K deficiency is more common than it was in previous
generations, the most likely explanation is the overuse of antibiotics
during the past several decades. As mentioned previously, much of
our vitamin K requirement is satisfied by vitamin K–producing intestinal bacteria. When you take an antibiotic, particularly a broad-
spectrum antibiotic such as tetracycline or a cephalosporin, you will
probably destroy some of your friendly intestinal bacteria. These

bacteria will not automatically return, once you have finished taking the antibiotic. On the contrary, unwanted bacteria or yeast may flourish and may compete effectively against your normal intestinal flora. In many cases, routine stool cultures identify organisms that the textbooks say do not belong in the intestinal tract. While ingestion of a high fiber diet and supplementation with garlic and acidophilus may help restore friendly organisms to the intestinal tract, we have no guarantee that intestinal vitamin K production today is the same as it was in the preantibiotic era.

ASSURING ADEQUATE INTAKE

Making sure you get adequate vitamin K from your diet is therefore extremely important. The major source of this vitamin is dark green leafy vegetables. As an added insurance policy, you may wish to supplement your diet with vitamin K. A reasonable dose is 150 to 500 mcg/day. Some multiple-vitamin and mineral formulas, particularly those designed for osteoporosis prevention, provide vitamin K in that dosage range. However, many nutritional supplements do not contain vitamin K, while others provide relatively insignificant amounts, such as 25 mcg/day. Although vitamin K toxicity can occur with very large intakes, the amounts we are discussing here are perfectly safe. Vitamin K toxicity has not been reported in adults taking less than 50 mg/day. That amount is 100 times greater than the highest daily dose I am recommending for supplementation (500 mcg is equivalent to 0.5 mg). For best absorption, vitamin K should probably be ingested along with a meal. Do not take vitamin K if you are taking coumadin or warfarin, since the vitamin interferes with the effect of these drugs.

NOTES

1. Gallop, P. M., J. B. Lian, and P. V. Hauschka. 1980. Carboxylated calcium-binding proteins and vitamin K. *N Engl J Med* 302:1460–1466.
2. Hart, J. P., et al. 1985. Electrochemical detection of depressed circulating levels of vitamin K1 in osteoporosis. *J Clin Endocrinol Metab* 60:1268–1269.

3. Robert D., et al. 1985. Hypercalciuria during experimental vitamin K deficiency in the rat. *Calcif Tissue Int* 37:143–147.

4. Tomita, A. 1971. Postmenopausal osteoporosis [47]Ca kinetic study with vitamin K2. *Clin Endocrinol* (Japan) 19:731–736. Article in Japanese (summary taken from review by P. M. Gallop). 1980. *N Engl J Med* 302:1460–1466.

5. Knapen, M. H. J., K. Hamulyak, and C. Vermeer. 1989. The effect of vitamin K supplementation on circulating osteocalcin (bone GLA protein) and urinary calcium excretion. *Ann Intern Med* 111:1001–1005.

6. The alternative explanation, that the increased urinary calcium excretion in postmenopausal women was due to excessive intestinal calcium absorption, is unlikely, since changes in urinary hydroxyproline excretion (a marker of bone turnover) paralleled the changes in urinary calcium. In addition, vitamin K supplementation does not appear to affect intestinal calcium absorption.

7. Bouckaert, J. H., and A. H. Said. 1960. Fracture healing by vitamin K. *Nature* 185:849. (*Note:* We appreciate the knowledge derived from the suffering of these animals, while acknowledging that they were not given a choice of whether to participate in the experiment.)

8. Bitensky, L., et al. 1988. Circulating vitamin K levels in patients with fractures. *J Bone Joint Surg* 70B:663–664.

4

Manganese

Manganese is the fourth most abundant biological trace element in the earth's crust and is found, although at relatively low concentrations, in most tissues of the body. The highest concentrations of manganese are in bone and in various endocrine glands. Manganese is known to be an essential nutrient for animals and circumstantial evidence suggests it is also essential for humans.

BASKETBALL BONES

Interest in the possibility that manganese deficiency may be one of the important factors related to the current epidemic of osteoporosis was stimulated by a rather unusual medical problem suffered by Bill Walton, a former NBA player.[1,2] After an illustrious college-playing career, Walton was considered one of the top "big men" in the game in the National Basketball Association. However, his future as a basketball player was in doubt because he seemed to suffer one fracture after another. During his basketball career, Walton had broken several fingers and toes, a cheek, a wrist, a leg, and his nose;

some more than once. In April, 1978, as a member of the Portland
Trail Blazers, he broke the tarsal navicular bone above the arch of
his left foot. Shortly thereafter, another crack developed in the same
bone. For reasons no one seemed to understand, the bone in his
foot refused to heal. When additional X rays were taken to evaluate
the poorly healing fracture, Walton's doctor was astonished to find
that his patient was suffering from osteoporosis. This was certainly
an unexpected finding in someone like Walton. This was not a
sedentary postmenopausal woman, the type of individual in whom
osteoporosis would be expected. Here was a young male, an accomplished athlete, in whom severe bone loss was the last thing the
doctor would have been looking for.

Perplexed by this unusual situation, Walton's physician consulted Paul Saltman, a biologist from the University of California, San
Diego. Saltman considered the possibility that nutritional deficiencies might be at the root of Walton's repeated fractures. After all, the
basketball star had for some time been consuming a macrobiotic
diet which has, in some instances, been known to cause various
vitamin and mineral deficiencies. Saltman therefore sent a sample
of Walton's blood serum to the lab to measure the concentrations
of manganese and other minerals. The report showed that the level
of copper was approximately 50% below normal and that zinc was
less than one-third of normal. Most surprising, however, was a complete absence of manganese in the blood, or at least not enough to
be detected by the instruments available at the time. Interestingly,
the concentration of calcium in the blood was increased, a finding
which suggested bone formation was being impaired. In other
words, the calcium was staying in the bloodstream, rather than being used to mineralize bone.

In an attempt to promote more effective bone healing, Walton
discontinued his macrobiotic diet and was given a supplement containing manganese, zinc, copper, calcium, magnesium, phosphorus,
fluoride, and iron. Within three days, the pain in his foot had improved and in eight weeks he was playing regularly for the first time
in nearly two seasons. He played more basketball in the early
months of 1980 than he had in the previous year and a half. After
he had been following this program for some time, the X rays were

repeated and his bones were found to be denser than before he had taken the supplements and changed his diet. Evidently, bone re-modeling and repair are in part dependent on manganese.

Bill Walton's dramatic improvement in bone health led re-searchers to pursue the manganese–osteoporosis connection further. In a study of fourteen Belgian women with osteoporosis, blood levels of manganese were 75% lower than those of women the same age without osteoporosis. To investigate the possibility that these low manganese levels were a reflection of generalized malnutrition, rather than specific to manganese, twenty-four other factors were also measured. However, of these measurements, the only statistically significant difference between the osteoporotic women and the control group was the level of manganese.[3] These observations suggest that manganese deficiency is common in in-dividuals with osteoporosis and that this deficiency may be one of the important factors that cause or aggravate bone loss.

MANGANESE INFLUENCES BONE HEALTH

Additional studies in both animals and humans provide evidence that manganese plays an important role in bone health. In rats fed a manganese-deficient diet, there was a reduction in the amount of calcium in the femur bone, indicating that manganese deficiency caused the bones to be thinner than normal.[4] Manganese deficiency also made the rats' bones more susceptible to breaking as a result of physical trauma.[5]

Manganese stimulates the production of a group of proteinlike molecules in bones called *mucopolysaccharides*.[6,7] These com-pounds provide a structure upon which calcification can take place. If the formation of mucopolysaccharides is impaired by manganese deficiency, then the process of calcification (and consequently, bone formation, remodeling, and repair) will be impaired.

OTHER EFFECTS OF DEFICIENCY

Manganese deficiency affects both humans and animals. Feed-ing animals a diet deficient in manganese results in a number of

abnormalities, including defective bone formation, impaired reproductive function, neurologic changes, damage to the insulin-
producing cells in the pancreas, and diabetes. Birds are particularly
suspectible to manganese deficiency. If deprived of adequate manganese intake, birds develop abnormal growth plates in the bones,
shortening and thickening of the bones, and abnormalities of the
Achilles' tendons.

Subtle deficiency of manganese may also be a factor contributing to the epidemic of cardiovascular disease in this country. In one
study, rabbits were fed a high-cholesterol diet to induce atherosclerosis (hardening of the arteries). When their diet was also supplemented with 10 mg of manganese, the extent of the atherosclerosis
was significantly reduced.[8]

Unlike scurvy, pellagra, and rickets, caused by deficiencies of
vitamins C, B3, and D, respectively, there is no *clearly* defined condition in humans that has been proven to be caused by manganese
deficiency. One possible consequence of manganese deficiency in
humans was suggested by observations on five patients with Down's
syndrome (also called mongolism). Each patient had an abnormality of one of their hips. The level of manganese in the hair of each
of these patients was extremely low, suggesting they were deficient
in this mineral. Since manganese deficiency causes similar abnormalities of the bones and joints in animals, it is quite possible that
the hip problems in these individuals were caused, at least in part,
by manganese deficiency.[9] There is also evidence that a particular
type of arthritis might be caused by a deficiency of manganese. A
condition, labeled Mseleni joint disease, affects 39% of the females
and 11% of the males in the Mseleni area of KwaZulu in South Africa,
a region thought to have a severe deficiency of manganese in the
soil and water.[10]

While a manganese deficiency severe enough to cause this
type of arthritis probably does not occur in other geographical
regions, one cannot rule out the possibility that subtle manganese
deficiency contributes to bone and joint disease in Western cultures. According to Carl C. Pfeiffer, M.D., current farming techniques deplete manganese from the soil, resulting in lower
concentrations of manganese in food. But since many crops can

flourish and appear perfectly healthy without manganese, a deficiency of manganese in food may not be suspected.[11] In addition, individuals who consume refined grains (such as white bread) obtain only about half as much manganese in their diet as those who eat whole grains. Thus, the typical American diet may not contain enough of this trace mineral.

WHAT CAUSES MANGANESE DEFICIENCY?

Environmental Pollutants

Why does manganese deficiency appear to be so common in people with osteoporosis? Although we cannot answer that question with certainty, there are several possible explanations. First, as mentioned previously, farming techniques and food processing may have reduced the amount of manganese we ingest every day. In addition, some of the pesticides, herbicides, preservatives, coloring agents, and other additives that contaminate our food supply may somehow interfere with the absorption or utilization of manganese. In my book *The Doctor's Guide to Vitamin B6,* I pointed out that chemicals present in our environment and in our food supply are known or suspected to interfere with both vitamin B6 and zinc.[12] The same may be true for manganese.

For example, ethylenediaminetetraacetic acid (EDTA), a preservative used in a number of different foods, is known to bind tightly to manganese.[13] It is probable, therefore, that EDTA inhibits the absorption of manganese. In addition, there may be an interaction between manganese and cadmium, a toxic element. One study found that manganese supplementation reduced the toxic effects of cadmium administered to rats.[14] This pervasive pollutant may also be draining our body stores of manganese. Although I am unaware of links between manganese and other food additives or environmental pollutants, I would be surprised if none of the tens of thousands of chemicals with which we are being bombarded have an adverse influence on our manganese status.

Inadequate Mineral Supplements

Another factor that might contribute to manganese deficiency is the use of mineral supplements that do not provide enough manganese. There is evidence that taking iron, magnesium, or calcium supplements may inhibit the uptake of manganese.[15] Many people, in the hope of preventing osteoporosis, take a calcium supplement, or calcium combined with magnesium, but do not back it up with other minerals. To the extent that calcium and magnesium interfere with manganese absorption, the beneficial effect of these minerals on bone health will be counterbalanced by a reduction in manganese status. That may be why administration of calcium alone has, in some studies, had absolutely no impact on osteoporosis (see Chapter 12). Many multiple vitamin and mineral supplements provide either no manganese at all or only a token amount of this important trace mineral (less than 1 mg). Roger Williams, Ph.D., a pioneer in nutritional medicine, reminded us that nutrients are found together in nature and work in the body as a team. In order for us to have a chance to achieve optimal health, we need adequate amounts of every essential nutrient, not just some of them. In our search for "magic bullets" to relieve us of our ailments, we often forget this simple principle of nutritional medicine.

Genetics

In addition to dietary factors and environmental exposures, our susceptibility to manganese deficiency may also have a genetic component. It is interesting to note that Bill Walton's aunt was also found to have manganese deficiency. Dr. Williams introduced the concept of biochemical individuality to argue that there are wide variations in nutritional needs among the human population. It is generally assumed that the variation in nutrient requirements is scattered into a bell-shaped curve; in other words, some people, for example, might need a little more vitamin C, while others can get by with a little less. However, for some individuals the requirement for one or more nutrients may lie far outside of that curve. Williams postulated that some people become ill because their genetic make-up causes them to need a lot more of a nutrient than they are able to obtain in their diet. In earlier times, when there was probably much more manganese in the diet, it was easier for people to obtain as much of this trace mineral as they needed. Today, however, those who have a higher than average need for manganese are more likely to show signs of deficiency.

Studies in animals have confirmed the hypothesis that susceptibility to manganese deficiency is inherited.[16] Perhaps this genetic variation in manganese requirements may explain in part why osteoporosis is a hereditary condition.

OBTAINING ENOUGH MANGANESE

Anyone interested in preventing osteoporosis should therefore make an effort to consume adequate amounts of this important mineral. Foods rich in manganese include whole grains, nuts, seeds, leafy vegetables, and meat. Manganese present in sugar cane is largely removed when it is processed into refined sugar. Similarly, most of the manganese in wheat is present in the germ portion; about 50% of the manganese is lost when whole wheat is refined to white flour.[17] Thus, diets high in sugar and white flour would tend to be low in manganese. The average diet contains about 3 to 9 mg of manganese per day. The optimal intake of manganese is not known, but it seems logical to recommend intakes toward the higher, rather than the lower, end of that range. Because manganese is inexpensive and nontoxic (at low doses), and because a little bit of extra manganese may go a long way toward preventing osteoporosis, I recommend that manganese be included as part of a comprehensive nutritional program.

High-quality multiple-vitamin and mineral supplements usually provide 5 to 25 mg of manganese per day. Although there are no well-defined guidelines for proper dosing of manganese, I usually recommend supplements that contain about 15 to 20 mg. That dosage level is somewhat of a compromise: probably enough to correct most deficiencies, but not too much to risk toxicity.

For those who prefer a natural source of manganese, rice

polish (or rice bran) is probably the best. Brown rice, which contains the bran component of the grain is also a good source, but white rice is not because the bran has been removed. Rice polish is also rich in silicon, another nutrient which appears to play a role in prevention of osteoporosis (see Chapter 11).

MANGANESE TOXICITY

Although manganese as a nutritional supplement is generally considered safe, the possibility of causing manganese poisoning must be kept in mind.[18,19,20] To date, manganese toxicity has been described exclusively in miners of manganese ore and in people working in steel mills who inhale manganese ore dust. Early symptoms of manganese poisoning are psychiatric in nature, and include disorientation, memory loss, anxiety, emotional lability, hallucinations, and delusions. These problems are followed later on by neurologic signs, which resemble Parkinson's disease to some extent. In some cases, manganese poisoning causes permanent damage to the brain.

The amount of manganese necessary to cause toxicity is not known. It is probable that the quantity that manganese-toxic workers introduced into their bodies was far more than anyone could obtain from a supplement. However, some nutritional products marketed for spinal disc problems contain very large amounts of manganese. It is possible by using these products to ingest hundreds of milligrams of manganese per day. While some practitioners are convinced that these high doses are beneficial and necessary, the potential for toxicity with long-term use must be borne in mind. Fortunately, there have been no reports so far of manganese toxicity from taking nutritional supplements.

CONCLUSION

In summary, the evidence suggests that the manganese content of modern diets is lower than in previous generations; that adulteration of our food and pollution of our environment may be interfering with absorption or utilization of manganese; and that some individuals have a higher need for manganese than others. As a result, manganese deficiency may be a common occurrence today, and may be a significant factor contributing to the increasing incidence of osteoporosis.

NOTES

1. Raloff, J. 1986. Reasons for boning up on manganese. *Science News* 130(27 Sept):199.
2. Gold, M. 1980. Basketball bones. *Science* 80 (May/June):101–102.
3. Raloff, 199.
4. Strause, L., and P. Saltman. 1985. Biochemical changes in rat skeleton following long-term dietary manganese and copper deficiencies. *Fed Proc* 44:752.
5. Amdur, M. O., L. C. Norris, and G. F. Heuser. 1945. The need for manganese in bone development by the rat. *Proc Soc Exp Biol Med* 59:254–255.
6. Leach, R. M., Jr., A-M. Muenster, E. M. Wien. 1969. Studies on the role of manganese in bone formation. II. Effect upon chondroitin sulfate synthesis in chick epiphyseal cartilage. *Arch Biochem Biophys* 133:22–28.
7. Ibid.
8. Bomb, B. S., et al. 1987. Regression of experimental atherosclerosis with manganese. *J Assoc Physicians India* 35:37.
9. Barlow, P. J., and P. E. Sylvester. 1983. Hip dislocation and manganese deficiency. *Lancet* 2:685.
10. Anonymous. 1981. Mseleni joint disease—a manganese deficiency? *S Afr Med J* 60:445–447.
11. Pfeiffer, C. C. 1978. *Zinc and other micro-nutrients.* New Canaan: Keats, p. 69.
12. Gaby, A. R. 1984, *The doctor's guide to vitamin B6.* Emmaus, Pa.: Rodale Press.
13. Cook, D. G., S. Fahn, and K. A. Brait. 1974. Chronic manganese intoxication. *Arch Neurol* 30:59–64.
14. Goering, P. L., and C. D. Klaassen. 1985. Mechanism of manganese-induced tolerance to cadmium lethality and hepatotoxicity. *Biochem Pharmacol* 34:1371–1379.
15. Raloff, 199.
16. Hurley, L. S., and L. T. Bell. Genetic influence on response to dietary manganese deficiency in mice. *J Nutr* 104:133–137.
17. Wenlock, R. W., D. H. Buss, and E. J. Dixon. 1979. Trace nutrients. 2. Manganese in British food. *Br J Nutr* 41:253–261.
18. Rosenstock, H. A., D. G. Simons, and J. S. Meyer. 1971. Chronic manganism.

Neurologic and laboratory studies during treatment with levodopa. *JAMA* 217:1354–1358.

19. Cook, Fahn, and Brait, 59–64.
20. Mena, I. 1974. The role of manganese in human disease. *Ann Clin Lab Sci* 4:487–491.

5

Magnesium: The Mineral That "Does It All"

Hardly a patient leaves my office without receiving a recommendation to take magnesium supplements. Magnesium is an essential mineral involved in more than fifty different biochemical reactions. As a cofactor in the production of ATP, the body's basic unit of stored energy, magnesium participates in all energy-dependent processes that take place in the body.

Magnesium deficiency appears to be extremely common, considering the wide range of different symptoms and conditions that improve with magnesium supplementation. A typical American diet contains only about 250 mg of magnesium/day, substantially less than the Recommended Dietary Allowance of 350 mg/day. The extent of magnesium deficiency may be even greater than these numbers suggest, since some researchers believe that the optimal daily intake of this mineral is more than 600 mg. Various kinds of physical, emotional, and chemical stresses are known to deplete magnesium, probably by causing the release of adrenaline, which draws magnesium out of the cells, allowing it to be flushed out in the urine. Animal studies have shown that something as simple as excessive noise can result in magnesium being lost from the body. Other factors that may promote magnesium deficiency include chronic diarrhea, excess alcohol consumption, and the use of certain prescription drugs, including some diuretics (hydrochlorothiazide, chlorthalidone, furosemide), digoxin (a heart drug), and cisplatinum (a cancer medication).

THERAPEUTIC USES OF MAGNESIUM

Research has shown magnesium to be effective in the prevention and treatment of a wide range of conditions. Furthermore, some of the beneficial effects of magnesium are among the most dramatic ever achieved in clinical medicine.

Heart Attacks

Magnesium therapy has proven to be life saving during the acute stages of a heart attack. In a recent study done in Israel and published in the *American Journal of Cardiology,* 103 patients hospitalized with suspected acute myocardial infarction were given either magnesium intravenously or a placebo, beginning as soon as possible after the patient arrived at the hospital.[1] The in-hospital death rate was 17% in the placebo group, compared to only 2% in the magnesium group, a reduction in mortality of 88.2%. No other treatment currently available has produced such a marked improvement in the death rate from myocardial infarction. A Dutch study published in the British medical journal *Lancet* in 1986 reported similar results with magnesium therapy.[2]

Asthma Attacks

Magnesium given intravenously has also been shown to relieve asthma attacks that had not responded to conventional treatment. In many cases, shortness of breath and wheezing improved within minutes after the magnesium was given.[3] For about eight years, I have given magnesium intravenously, combined with calcium,

B-vitamins, and vitamin C to treat asthma attacks. This treatment usually relieves the asthma within a minute or two, saving the patient a trip to the emergency room and possible hospitalization. Furthermore, this injection is not only inexpensive, but virtually free of side effects. This combination of injected nutrients was popularized by the late John Myers, M.D., of Baltimore, Maryland, whose patients taught it to me after his death.

Other Therapeutic Uses

I have used a modification of the "Myers' cocktail" with great success for other conditions, including chronic fatigue, depression, fibromyalgia (a common condition which causes muscle pain and spasm), chronic urticaria (hives), congestive heart failure, angina, and acute infections. I have presented information on intravenous nutrient therapy at medical seminars during the past eight years, and I estimate that more than one thousand physicians are currently making use of this treatment. A brief discussion of the indications and administration of intravenous nutrients is presented in Appendix A.

Numerous other uses for magnesium have been documented in medical journals, including treatment of chronic fatigue, premenstrual syndrome, high blood pressure, cardiac arrhythmias (heart rhythm abnormalities), epilepsy, diabetes, reactive hypoglycemia, and prevention of alcohol withdrawal symptoms. Magnesium supplements have also been found to reduce the recurrence rate of kidney stones by more than 90% in chronic stone formers. In combination with vitamin B6, magnesium has also been used with some success to treat autistic children.

MAGNESIUM AND OSTEOPOROSIS

As much as 50% of all the magnesium in the body is found in the bones. It should not be surprising, therefore, that studies have demonstrated a role for magnesium in the prevention and treatment of osteoporosis. Israeli scientists measured magnesium status in nineteen osteoporotic women by means of a magnesium load test. In that test, a standard amount of magnesium is given intravenously and the urine is collected over the next twenty-four hours. If most of the magnesium is excreted in the urine, then, by inference, the body did not need the extra amount. If, on the other hand, most of the magnesium is retained by the body, then the individual is presumed to have a magnesium deficiency. The reason this type of test is used to assess magnesium status is that blood magnesium levels and other readily available measurements are unreliable.

Of the nineteen women who received the intravenous magnesium load, sixteen retained about 90%, indicating significant magnesium deficiency. Interestingly, magnesium status appeared to have a major influence on the type of calcium crystals present in the bones of these women. Of the sixteen women who had evidence of magnesium deficiency, every one had abnormally large calcium crystals, the shapes of which were also abnormal. On the other hand, each of the three women with adequate magnesium status had normal crystals. This study demonstrates that magnesium deficiency is common in women with osteoporosis and is associated with abnormal calcification of bone.[4]

This abnormality of calcification in the bones of magnesium-deficient women may be one of the factors that increases fracture risk. As noted previously, not all women with reduced bone mineral content develop fractures. Why are some women with thin bones protected, while others break their bones easily? It is likely that the quality of the bone is as important as the quantity. Just as a thin crowbar can withstand more stress than a thin piece of chalk, so it is that well-formed bone crystals would provide more resistance and resiliency than improperly formed crystals. The amount of magnesium is probably one of the factors determining how strong your bones will be.

TRIAL OF MAGNESIUM THERAPY

Because of the evidence that magnesium is important in osteoporosis, Guy E. Abraham, M.D., conducted a trial of magnesium therapy in twenty-six postmenopausal women who were recruited from a menopause clinic.[5] All the women were taking either estrogen alone or estrogen plus a progestogen. The women were given dietary advice, including (1) avoid processed foods, (2) limit protein intake; emphasize vegetable protein over animal protein, and (3) limit the consumption of refined sugar, salt, alcohol, coffee, tea, chocolate, and tobacco. Each participant was also offered a daily supplement containing 500 mg of calcium (citrate) and 600 mg of magnesium (oxide). The supplement also contained vitamin C, B-vitamins, vitamin D, zinc, copper, manganese, boron, and other nutrients. Nineteen women took the supplement, while seven chose not to. Bone density studies were performed on the calcaneous bone (a bone in the foot), both before and an average of 8 to 9 months after treatment was begun. In the women who did not take the supplement, average bone density increased slightly, by 0.7%. However, in those who did take the supplement, the results were dramatically better—an average increase in bone density of 11%.

An 11% increase in bone mineral density in a period of 8 to 9 months is astounding. With the exception of the report by John Lee, M.D., on natural progesterone therapy (see Chapter 15), no other studies have come close to achieving that level of improvement in so short a period of time. In the early postmenopausal period, untreated women typically *lose* 3 to 8% of their bone mass per year. In those who receive estrogen replacement therapy with a progestogen, bone loss may be slowed down or actually reversed to some extent. In Abraham's study, hormone replacement therapy alone (the control group) produced a small (0.7%) increase in bone density. But that slight improvement was nothing, compared to the 11% increase in the diet–hormone–nutritional supplement group.

What the Results Mean

In his discussion of the results, Dr. Abraham attributed the improvements to the large quantity of magnesium in his supplement. However, that explanation is probably only partially correct. While it is certainly possible that a higher than normal dose of magnesium could exert an added bone-building effect, it is also likely that the other aspects of Abraham's treatment contributed to the superior results. Abraham's program included not only magnesium, but broad dietary recommendations, and a comprehensive list of other vitamins and minerals. Most of the diet changes and supplements Abraham provided are discussed in this book as being of possible value for prevention of osteoporosis.

While we should not minimize the value of magnesium, Abraham's results are most likely due to the combined effect of many different interventions. For example, there is evidence that vitamin C, B-vitamins, vitamin D, zinc, copper, manganese, and boron each exert beneficial effects on bone. The lifestyle changes recommended by Abraham, particularly avoiding sugar, caffeine, alcohol, and to-bacco, may have produced additional benefit. Abraham's dramatic results tend to validate the thesis of this book: that a comprehensive program of lifestyle modification, nutritional supplementation, and judicious hormone therapy holds the most promise in the battle against osteoporosis. While an 11% gain in bone mass in 8 to 9 months is certainly impressive, such results might be even further improved if some of the other interventions discussed in this book are used.

Although the results of hormone therapy by itself (the control group) were not particularly impressive, it is possible that the effects of lifestyle change and nutritional supplementation are greater when hormones are also being used than when they are not. In addition, as suggested in Chapter 15, the results of hormone therapy may be better when natural progesterone is used instead of a syn-thetic progestogen.

OBTAINING ENOUGH MAGNESIUM

In summary, there are many reasons that you should try to get enough magnesium in your diet, not the least of which is prevention of osteoporosis. Foods rich in magnesium include whole grains, nuts and seeds, green vegetables, and animal foods. Sugars and fats contain virtually no magnesium, and about 80% of the magnesium is lost when whole grain flour is refined to make white flour. Consumption of too much alcohol can also deplete your magnesium. A diet that emphasizes whole foods will increase your chances of obtaining enough magnesium. Because this nutrient is so critical in so many different ways, and because supplementation is safe and inexpensive, I advise nearly all of my patients to take a magnesium supplement or a multiple vitamin and mineral formula that contains magnesium. A reasonable dose is 250 to 600 mg per day. It should be noted that many of the one-tablet-per-day vitamin and mineral supplements contain very little magnesium, because this mineral takes up a lot of room in a tablet. Multiple-nutrient supplements that contain enough magnesium are generally those that recommend between three and six tablets per day. It should also be pointed out that too much magnesium may cause loose bowels in some people. Furthermore, individuals with renal failure should not take magnesium without medical supervision.

NOTES

1. Shechter, M., et al. 1990. Beneficial effect of magnesium sulfate in acute myocardial infarction. *Am J Cardiol* 66:271–274.

2. Rasmussen, H. S., et al. 1986. Intravenous magnesium in acute myocardial infarction. *Lancet* 1:234–236.

3. Okayama, H., et al. 1987. Bronchodilating effect of intravenous magnesium sulfate in bronchial asthma. *JAMA* 257:1076–1078.

4. Cohen, L., and R. Kitzes. 1981. Infrared spectroscopy and magnesium content of bone mineral in osteoporotic women. *Isr J Med Sci* 17:1123–1125.

5. Abraham, G. E., and H. Grewal. 1990. A total dietary program emphasizing magnesium instead of calcium. Effect on the mineral density of calcaneous bone in postmenopausal women on hormonal therapy. *J Reprod Med* 35:503–507.

6

Folic Acid

Folic acid is one of the members of the B-vitamin group. It was given its name by nutritionist Roger Williams, Ph.D., because of its presence in high concentrations in leafy vegetables, or "foliage." This vitamin participates in many fundamental biochemical activities in the body. Folic acid deficiency is a well recognized cause of anemia, psychiatric symptoms, and neurologic damage. Adequate folic acid is also required for the immune system to function properly.

Folic acid deficiency is one of the most frequently encountered nutritional problems. Individuals who consume a diet low in vegetables are at risk for becoming deficient. In addition, because folic acid is a relatively unstable molecule that can be destroyed by heat or light, a large proportion of this vitamin may be lost when food is overcooked or processed. Individuals who drink excessive amounts of alcohol often become deficient in folic acid, because alcohol interferes with folic acid absorption and impairs the utilization of this vitamin in the body. Birth control pills, which are taken by more than 10 million American women, also have a tendency to cause folic acid deficiency. Other potential causes of folic acid deficiency include chronic diarrhea and use of the anticonvulsant drug dilantin. Doctors often prescribe folic acid to treat anemia and for various neurological or psychiatric symptoms associated with alcoholism.

NEURAL TUBE DEFECTS

A growing body of evidence also suggests that supplementing pregnant women with folic acid greatly reduces the chances of the baby being born with a neural tube defect, such as spina bifida or hydrocephalus.[1] The neural tube is that portion of the embryo that eventually develops into the brain and spinal cord. If the neural tube does not form properly, the infant may be born with severe and permanent neurological problems. Neural tube defects are among the most common birth defects, occurring in about 2 of every 1,000 live births. Research on folic acid and neural tube defects was originally met with skepticism within the medical community. However, more recent studies have firmly established that supplementing with folic acid before and during the early stages of pregnancy prevents both recurrences[2] and first occurrences[3] of neural tube defects. On the basis of this information, the United States Public Health Service released a statement on September 11, 1992, recommending that "all women of childbearing age in the United States who are capable of becoming pregnant should consume 0.4 mg of folic acid per day for the purpose of reducing their risk of having a pregnancy affected with spina bifida or other NTD's [neural tube defects]."[4]

ABNORMAL PAP SMEARS

Another use for folic acid is for preventing or treating cervical dysplasia (the medical term for the precancerous changes seen on Pap smears). Twenty years ago it was reported that women taking birth control pills frequently developed abnormal Pap smears, described as megaloblastic changes in the cervical epithelium (the cells lining the cervix). These abnormalities disappeared after the women were treated with large doses of folic acid (10 mg/day) for three weeks. The authors of the study suggested that oral contraceptives cause a localized interference with folic acid metabolism in the cells of the cervix.[5]

This original report was followed up by C. E. Butterworth, Jr., M.D., and associates from the Department of Nutrition Sciences of the University of Alabama School of Medicine. In a double-blind study of forty-seven women with mild or moderate cervical dysplasia who were taking oral contraceptives, treatment with 10 mg/day of folic acid for three months produced a significant improvement in the results of the Pap smears.[6] Butterworth's study suggested one of two possibilities: (1) that a localized deficiency of folic acid may sometimes be misdiagnosed as cervical dysplasia, or (2) that cervical dysplasia is caused in part by localized folic acid deficiency and can be prevented or reversed by folic acid supplementation.

The second possibility was supported by an exciting new study by Butterworth and colleagues, published in the *Journal of the American Medical Association*.[7] In that study, the effect of human papilloma virus (HPV-16), a common sexually transmitted infection, on cervical dysplasia was determined. In women who had evidence of folic acid deficiency (red blood cell folic acid levels at or below 660 nmol/L), infection with HPV-16 increased the risk of developing cervical dysplasia by more than fivefold. However, in women whose folic acid levels were above that cutoff point, the presence of HPV-16 did not seem to increase the risk of cervical dysplasia at all. Stated differently, maintaining adequate folic acid status may prevent the damaging effects of a common sexually transmitted disease.

HEALING DISEASED GUMS

Folic acid has also been shown to be of value in the treatment of gingivitis (inflammation of the gums), also known as periodontal disease. In one study, sixty individuals with gingivitis received a mouthwash containing a 0.1% folic acid solution or a placebo mouthwash. Each volunteer used 1 teaspoon of the mouthwash twice a day, rinsing it in the mouth for one minute and then spitting it out. After four weeks, the improvement in gingival health was significantly greater in the folic acid group than in the placebo group.[8] In a second study, folic acid was swallowed, instead of being applied directly as a mouth rinse. Thirty patients received either 4 mg/day of folic acid or a placebo, in a double-blind study. After 30 days, there was a significant reduction in gingival inflammation in the folic acid group, but not in the placebo group.[9] The results of these two studies suggest that localized folic acid deficiency plays a role in the development of gingivitis, even if folic acid levels in the bloodstream are normal. Direct application of folic acid or oral administration of larger than normal doses of the vitamin can saturate the deficient tissues and reverse gingival inflammation.

THE RATIONALE FOR NUTRIENT SUPPLEMENTATION

The possibility that the level of a nutrient can be abnormally low in one tissue or compartment of the body, but adequate throughout the rest of the system, is a foreign concept to many physicians. Nevertheless, the evidence just presented suggests that folic acid deficiency does occur in specific tissues (for example, cervical epithelium and gingival tissue), even if blood tests for folic acid are normal. There are actually many situations in which localized deficiencies have been documented. For example, heart disease is frequently accompanied by magnesium deficiency in the heart muscle, but normal magnesium levels in the blood serum.[10] Some elderly individuals who suffer from dementia have unusually low concentrations of vitamin B12 in their brain, but normal amounts of this vitamin in their blood.[11] If blood tests are relied upon to diagnose tissue-specific deficiencies, then a lot of clinically important deficiencies will be missed.

OSTEOPOROSIS: THE
HOMOCYSTEINE CONNECTION

I have discussed the existence of tissue-specific deficiencies to introduce the possibility that folic acid supplements may help prevent osteoporosis, even if blood levels of this vitamin are normal. Studies indicate that certain changes occur in a woman's metabolism around the time of menopause. These changes cause a harmful compound that probably contributes to accelerated postmenopausal bone loss to build up in the body. Research suggests that this process can be prevented or inhibited by supplementing with folic acid.

This potentially damaging substance is called *homocysteine,* a breakdown product of methionine, one of the essential amino acids. *Methionine,* a component of the protein we ingest from food, is one of the building blocks used by the body to manufacture its own proteins. In the normal course of metabolism, some of the methionine in the body is broken down to homocysteine which is, in turn, converted either back to methionine or to other compounds. There is evidence that homocysteine is harmful; perhaps that is why the body contains several different biochemical pathways by which homocysteine can be eliminated. The problem is that these pathways do not always function efficiently and, consequently, homocysteine levels can build up under certain circumstances.

The damage that homocysteine can do to the human body is illustrated by a genetic disorder called *homocystinuria,* in which homocysteine builds up to unusually high levels in the body. Individuals with homocystinuria frequently develop atherosclerosis (hardening of the arteries) and osteoporosis as early as age twenty.

MENOPAUSE AFFECTS
HOMOCYSTEINE METABOLISM

To review what we have said so far, homocysteine is a breakdown product of methionine. Homocysteine has the potential to promote atherosclerosis and osteoporosis if the body does not detoxify it efficiently. It is interesting to note that premenopausal women are largely protected from both of these diseases. However, after menopause, the risk of developing both cardiovascular disease and osteoporosis skyrockets. The onset of menopause is also associated with a reduced capacity to metabolize homocysteine. Is this change in homocysteine metabolism one of the reasons that postmenopausal women lose their protection against these diseases? If so, is there anything you can do about it?

A group of Swedish researchers, led by Lars E. Brattstrom, M.D., performed several experiments designed to shed light on these questions. Brattstrom found that fasting plasma homocysteine levels were significantly higher in postmenopausal than in premenopausal women. That finding suggests that something happens around the time of menopause that impairs the body's ability to break down homocysteine.

The Methionine Load Test

The difference in homocysteine metabolizing capacity between pre- and postmenopausal women was shown to be even more pronounced when a more sensitive test, the methionine load test, was used. A methionine load test is performed by measuring the rise in plasma homocysteine after ingesting methionine (100 mg per kg of body weight). After ingesting methionine, homocysteine concentrations in the postmenopausal women rose markedly and were considerably higher than they were in the premenopausal women. In fact, there was no overlap between the two groups of women. Clearly, then, homocysteine tends to build up in postmenopausal women. Furthermore, this accumulation of homocysteine is probably made worse by ingesting foods high in methionine, such as meat, chicken, fish, and eggs.

The Effects of Folic Acid

Because folic acid is involved in the breakdown of homocysteine, Brattstrom investigated whether supplementing with folic acid would prevent the rise in plasma homocysteine levels that happens after menopause. Each of the women in the study mentioned previously was given 5 mg of folic acid daily for four weeks, following which all of the measurements were repeated. In the postmenopausal women, folic acid therapy resulted in significant reductions in homocysteine levels, both before the methionine load (31% reduction) and after (28% reduction). These improvements occurred, even though pretreatment folic acid concentrations in the serum and red blood cells were completely normal. In other words, supplementing with folic acid produced an apparently beneficial effect, even though none of the women had any evidence of folic acid deficiency by standard laboratory tests. The authors of the study concluded that moderate elevations of homocysteine contribute to postmenopausal atherosclerosis and osteoporosis and that folic acid therapy might have a preventive effect.[12]

To confirm their original observations, Brattstrom and associates studied forty-two healthy men and women between the ages of 43 and 56 years. In this study, administering 5 mg/day of folic acid for fourteen days reduced the average plasma homocysteine concentration by 52%. Vitamin B6 (40 mg/day) and vitamin B12 (1,000 mcg/day) were also tried, since they are known to play a role in homocysteine metabolism. However, the only vitamin that had an effect on homocysteine levels was folic acid.[13]

The reason that homocysteine metabolism becomes less efficient after menopause is not known. Perhaps the decline in hormone levels affects the efficiency of certain enzymes that break down homocysteine. Whatever the reason, it seems that this potentially damaging substance can be kept in check by additional amounts of folic acid. And, based on what we know about homocysteine, keeping the levels down might help prevent osteoporosis.

HOW MUCH FOLIC ACID IS ENOUGH?

In Brattstrom's study, the dosage of folic acid was arbitrarily set at 5 mg/day. That level is more than twelve times the Recommended Dietary Allowance of 0.4 mg/day (400 mcg/day). We do not know whether that large a dose is necessary to achieve the desired effect. Surveys have shown that the American diet often provides less than 50% of the RDA for this vitamin.[14] On the other hand, low serum folic acid levels are relatively uncommon in healthy individuals. Perhaps all Brattstrom was doing was correcting a mild folic acid deficiency that was too subtle to show up on standard blood tests, but significant enough to affect homocysteine metabolism. If that is the case, then a relatively small increase in folic acid intake might be all that is needed. On the other hand, it is also possible that homocysteine metabolism can be further enhanced by providing even larger amounts of folic acid than 5 mg/day. Hopefully, additional research will answer these questions.

Homocysteine and Animal Protein

The amount of folic acid you need may depend in part on how much animal protein you consume. As mentioned, ingesting methionine causes the level of homocysteine in your body to rise. The major dietary sources of methionine are meat, chicken, fish, dairy products, and eggs. While methionine is an essential nutrient, many people in the United States consume more protein (and, consequently, more methionine) than they need. In addition to putting a strain on the kidneys, a diet high in animal protein places an extra burden on the body's homocysteine detoxifying mechanisms. If you eat more vegetarian dishes and less animal foods, you will have less homocysteine to deal with and, consequently, a lower risk of developing heart disease and osteoporosis.

USING FOLIC ACID WISELY AND SAFELY

Although folic acid is present in a wide variety of foods, the most highly concentrated source of this vitamin is fresh vegetables. Raw or lightly steamed vegetables provide a great deal more folic acid than overcooked or canned vegetables. Wheat germ and brewer's yeast are also good sources of folic acid. Unfortunately, though, even the best diet would not come close to providing 5 mg/day of folic acid. To obtain that amount, supplementation is necessary. Most multiple-vitamin formulas provide only 0.4 mg of folic acid; some supply 0.8 mg. Folic acid tablets are available in health food stores in doses of 0.4 and 0.8 mg, and by prescription in doses of 1 mg. A few nutrition-oriented pharmacies around the country carry 5 mg and 25 mg tablets.

Several precautions should be taken by anyone using large doses of folic acid. First, you should be aware that taking folic acid supplements will interfere with the screening test used to diagnose pernicious anemia (a relatively uncommon but serious condition caused by vitamin B12 malabsorption). Doctors may suspect the presence of pernicious anemia if certain abnormalities are found on a complete blood count. However, if you have pernicious anemia and are also taking a large amount of folic acid, the complete blood count may be normal, even while vitamin B12 deficiency is causing progressive and irreversible damage to your central nervous system. If you are planning to take more than 1 mg/day of folic acid, you should first have a complete blood count to screen for early signs of pernicious anemia. As an added precaution, it would be wise to measure your serum vitamin B12 level every two years, as long as you are taking large amounts of folic acid. This test will detect cases of pernicious anemia that may have been missed by a complete blood count. Since it takes three to five years for vitamin B12 deficiency to develop, it is not necessary to test your vitamin B12 level every year.

Second, you should be aware of the common drug and nutrient interactions with folic acid. There is some evidence that taking large doses of folic acid can interfere with the anticonvulsant drug dilantin, and might therefore cause a return of seizures in susceptible individuals. Although this interaction generally does not occur at folic acid doses below 15 mg/day, anyone taking dilantin should consult a physician before taking more than 1 mg/day of folic acid. Another consideration is that folic acid competes with zinc for intestinal absorption. Consequently, ingesting large doses of either zinc or folic acid could cause a deficiency of the other. If you are taking megadoses of either of these nutrients, you should also be taking at least some of the other. I am not aware of any good studies showing that these two nutrients must be taken at different times of the day. If you take these precautions, folic acid supplementation should be quite safe.

NOTES

1. Laurence, K. M., et al. 1981. Double-blind randomised controlled trial of folate treatment before conception to prevent recurrence of neural-tube defects. *Br Med J* 282:1509–1511.

2. MRC Vitamin Study Research Group. 1991. Prevention of neural tube defects: Results of the Medical Research Council vitamin study. *Lancet* 338:131–137.

3. Czeizel, A. E., and I. Dudas. 1992. Prevention of the first occurrence of neural-tube defects by periconceptional vitamin supplementation. *N Engl J Med* 327:1832–1835.

4. Rosenberg, I. H. 1992. Folic acid and neural-tube defects—time for action? *N Engl J Med* 327:1875–1877.

5. Whitehead, N., F. Reyner, and J. Lindenbaum. 1973. Megaloblastic changes in cervical epithelium: association with oral contraceptive therapy and reversal with folic acid. *JAMA* 226:1421–1424.

6. Butterworth, C. E., Jr., et al. 1982. Improvement in cervical dysplasia associated with folic acid therapy in users of oral contraceptives. *Am J Clin Nutr* 35:73–82.

7. Butterworth, C. E., Jr., et al. 1992. Folate deficiency and cervical dysplasia. *JAMA* 267:528–533.

8. Pack, A. R. C. 1984. Folate mouthwash: Effects on established gingivitis in periodontal patients. *J Clin Periodontol* 11:619–628.

9. Vogel, R. I., et al. 1976. The effect of folic acid on gingival health. *J Periodontol* 47:667–668.

10. Frustaci, A., et al. 1987. Myocardial magnesium content, histology, and antiarrhythmic response to magnesium infusion. *Lancet* 2:1019.

11. van Tiggelen, C. J. M., J. P. C. Peperkamp, and J. F. W. Tertoolen. 1983. Vitamin B12 levels of cerebrospinal fluid in patients with organic mental disorder. *J Orthomolec Psychiatry* 12:305.

12. Brattstrom, L. E., B. L. Hultberg, and J. E. Hardebo. 1985. Folic acid responsive postmenopausal homocysteinemia. *Metabolism* 34:1073–1077.

13. Brattstrom, L. E., et al. 1988. Folic acid—an innocuous means to reduce plasma homocysteine. *Scand J Clin Lab Invest* 48:215–221.

14. Daniel, W. A., Jr., E. G. Gaines, and D. L. Bennett. 1975. Dietary intakes and plasma concentrations of folate in healthy adolescents. *Am J Clin Nutr* 28:363–370.

7

Boron

Boron is the fifth element of the periodic table. It occurs in nature primarily as borax, a combination of boron, sodium, and oxygen. Borax has been known for centuries as a valuable cleaning agent, and was used medicinally by Arabian physicians more than one thousand years ago.[1] Boron compounds are also used as buffering agents in some medications, as water softeners, and in soaps, mouthwashes, enamel, pottery, and glass. Boric acid, synthesized from borax, is used as a mild antiseptic and in the production of cement.

The fact that boron is essential for plants has been recognized for a long time. A lack of boron in the soil will result in a variety of plant diseases, such as "top sickness" in tobacco, "brown-heart" in turnips, "cork-spot" in apples, and "heart-rot" in sugar beets.[2]

Until recently, boron was not thought to be essential for animals. However, studies during the past decade or so have demonstrated a role for this element in the nutrition of both animals and humans. In 1981, Forrest H. Nielsen, Ph.D., a biochemist at the Human Nutrition Research Center of the U.S. Department of

Agriculture, found that a diet deficient in both boron and vitamin D caused growth retardation and bone abnormalities in chickens.[3] While vitamin D deficiency alone caused these problems, they were made worse by simultaneous deficiency of boron. Further studies demonstrated that the requirement for boron was increased when the diet was low in magnesium and that a combined deficiency of magnesium and boron caused detrimental changes in bone.

OSTEOPOROSIS STUDY

Because boron appeared to influence bone health, Nielsen and coworkers studied the effect of boron on postmenopausal bone loss.[4] Twelve postmenopausal women, ages 48 to 82, were maintained on a diet low in boron for 119 days. The reduction in boron intake to 0.25 mg/day was accomplished by restricting fruits, vegetables, and nuts, the main dietary sources of this element. After 119 days, an additional 3 mg/day of boron was provided in supplement form. This extra supply of boron produced some rather remarkable changes in the body's metabolism—changes that appeared to be of great significance with respect to osteoporosis. First, boron supplementation reduced the urinary excretion of calcium by 44% and also reduced urinary magnesium excretion. Boron also markedly increased the serum concentrations of 17β-estradiol (the biologically active form of estrogen) and testosterone. In fact, the concentration of 17β-estradiol in boron-supplemented women was the same as that in women receiving estrogen replacement therapy. These dramatic findings suggested that boron has a powerful influence on the metabolism of calcium, magnesium, and some hormones, and that this trace element may be useful for preventing bone loss.

BIOCHEMICAL FUNCTION OF BORON

It is rare that a previously unknown nutritional element appears unexpectedly and is shown to exert such a powerful influence on metabolism and bone health. It may seem hard to believe that a substance that had heretofore completely escaped the notice of scientists and nutritionists could be found to affect so many different biochemical events. However, when one looks at the biochemistry of boron, its role in human and animal metabolism no longer seems farfetched.

Boron is known to form complexes with organic compounds that contain hydroxyl groups (a hydroxyl group is the combination of an oxygen and a hydrogen atom; the chemical symbol is –OH). The synthesis of certain hormones in the body from precursor molecules involves one or more hydroxylation steps (that is, the addition of an –OH group). Thus, the synthesis of both estrogen and testosterone, both of which involve hydroxylation reactions, might be enhanced in the human body by boron. It should not be surprising, then, that boron supplementation increased the levels of both of these hormones.

In addition, boron may also enhance the conversion of vitamin D to its biologically active hormonal form (1,25-dihydroxyvitamin D; a conversion that involves two hydroxylation reactions). In another study by Nielsen of human volunteers, supplementation of a low-boron diet with 3 mg/day of boron did, indeed, increase blood levels of a form of vitamin D.[5]

As discussed elsewhere in this book, each of these three hormones—estrogen, testosterone, and 1,25-dihydroxyvitamin D—plays a role in the prevention of bone loss. And, because boron may affect the metabolism of these hormones, it, too, could have an influence on the development of osteoporosis.

BORON REQUIREMENT

Nielsen has estimated, on the basis of animal studies, that the human requirement for boron is 1 to 2 mg/day. Diets that contain liberal amounts of fruits, vegetables, and nuts should provide at least that much boron. No one knows whether boron supplementation is valuable only when the diet is deficient, or whether amounts greater than the typical "requirement" would have an additional effect. In the Nielsen study described previously, the women were placed on a boron-deficient diet for nearly four months prior to receiving a small dose of boron. His study, therefore, measured only the effect of correcting a deficiency. Further studies are needed to assess the effect of boron supplementation in women who do not have an obvious deficiency.

Of course, as is the case with other nutrients, some people may absorb boron poorly, excrete it more rapidly than normal, or have some other genetic or acquired defect that would increase their nutritional requirement for boron. Since there has been little research so far on this interesting nutrient, we do not know for sure what the minimum requirement is, or whether that requirement differs significantly from the "optimal" level of intake. Until such work is done, we will have to rely on educated guesses.

Women who consult me for menopausal symptoms—hot flashes, vaginal dryness, depression, and so forth—frequently request a nutritional treatment because they are concerned about the risks of estrogen replacement therapy. My clinical observations indicate that boron is definitely not as effective as estrogen in relieving hot flashes, even though Nielsen's work found that boron raised estrogen levels substantially. Although an occasional patient has reported marked improvement in menopausal symptoms after taking boron supplements, most women have found only slight improvement or none at all.

IS BORON SAFE?

Boron and Cancer

Because of its ability to raise estrogen levels, and because estrogen promotes cancer under certain circumstances, the possibility that boron supplements might cause cancer must also be considered. However, several lines of reasoning strongly suggest that this is not the case. In the first place, epidemiologic studies indicate that diets high in fruits and vegetables (and, therefore, high in boron) decrease, rather than increase, the risk of cancer. While it is possible that other nutrients in these foods, such as beta-carotene, vitamin E, and folic acid, would counteract a proposed negative effect of boron, there are other reasons to believe that boron not only does not cause cancer, but may actually prevent it.

Again, boron is thought to participate in hydroxylation reactions (addition of an –OH group). In the metabolism of estrogen, the cancer-promoting forms of estrogen, estrone and estradiol, are hydroxylated to a noncancer-causing estrogen, called *estriol.* In fact, there is evidence that estriol actually *prevents* cancer.[6] As pointed out in Chapter 14, an imbalance between these hormones may be one of the factors determining whether or not estrogen will promote cancer. If a woman has too little estriol in her body, then the risk of developing breast cancer (and possibly other types of cancer) will be increased.[7] Since boron could increase the production of estriol, this mineral might decrease the risk of cancer. Women who have been diagnosed with breast cancer have been found to have a reduced capacity to hydroxylate estrogen molecules.[8] This defect may be correctable by supplementing with boron.

Another possible effect of boron that might reduce cancer risk is in relation to the adrenal steroid hormone dehydroepiandrosterone (DHEA). As discussed in Chapter 16, DHEA has a number of beneficial physiologic effects, including prevention of breast cancer and other types of cancer. DHEA is produced in the body from a hormone called *pregnenolone,* which is converted to 17-alpha-hydroxy-pregnenolone, and then to DHEA. As the chemical name suggests, the first step in this two-step conversion process is a hydroxylation reaction. Thus, the synthesis of DHEA, an important anticancer substance, may also depend in part on an adequate supply of boron.

The Need for More Boron Research

Much of this discussion is speculative. In medicine, however, we are often faced with making decisions on the basis of incomplete data. It would certainly help if more researchers were taking a serious look at the nutritional effects of boron. Unfortunately, there is no money to be made from a compound that is mined by the ton, but ingested only in milligram quantities. At a dosage of 3 mg/day, 1 ton of boron could supply a million women for nearly a year. Because there is no potential for profit, the pharmaceutical industry has had no interest in funding boron research.

Toxic Levels of Boron

It is certainly possible to kill yourself by swallowing a pound of borax; however, there appears to be a comfortable safety margin for boron in the nutritional dosage range. In chronic toxicity studies using dogs and rats, no adverse effects resulted from long-term administration of 350 parts per million of boron in the diet.[9] That dosage level corresponds to approximately 117 mg/day in humans, an amount far greater than the 1 to 3 mg/day being considered for nutritional supplementation. In certain parts of the world where the diet contains as much as 41 mg/day of boron, no unusual medical problems and no increase in cancer risk have been reported.[10]

TRYING "UNPROVEN" REMEDIES

In the day-by-day practice of medicine, doctors look for safe, effective, and inexpensive remedies for what ails their patients. We are also trained as scientists, to distinguish what is proven versus what is unproven. As a scientist, I would be the first to point out that boron is an unproven remedy for osteoporosis. As a physician looking out for the welfare of my patients, however, I have no qualms about recommending this safe and inexpensive, though unproven, substance. I suspect that some of the outspoken critics of nutritional medicine, the ones who chastise us for using "unproven" remedies, would try some of these treatments themselves if they became ill. On the other hand, they would probably be afraid to admit to their colleagues that they were doing so.

This discrepancy between the public position and the personal philosophy of doctors was poignantly illustrated by a recent report from the *Harvard Letter,* a medical newsletter written for the public. In a survey of the health and nutrition habits of 672 members of the clinical faculty of Harvard Medical School, 80% of the respondents reported that they either took beta-carotene supplements or maintained a high intake of beta-carotene through their diet. In addition, 23% of the respondents regularly took vitamin and mineral supplements. The editor called this 23% figure "surprisingly high . . . given the evidence that these items provide little or no benefit for healthy people consuming a balanced diet."[11]

This survey of Harvard doctors is relevant to the ongoing controversy that surrounds nutritional medicine. Based on the available data, many doctors have chosen to change their diet or to take nutritional supplements to enhance their own health. However, when it comes to making recommendations for their patients, they put their "dispassionate scientist" hat back on and refuse to take a stand. There is no doubt that some doctors are afraid of being ridiculed by their colleagues for recommending "unproven" treatments. There is also the very real threat of being disciplined by state medical peer review committees for deviating from the standards of care in the community.

So, something new and simple like boron comes along, something that common sense tells us should be tried, and the conventional medical community looks the other way and pretends it does not exist. The same scenario has occurred with dozens of other simple, safe, and inexpensive natural remedies. The medical establishment hides behind the allegation that "alternative medicine" is unproven, even though a fair reading of the medical literature clearly shows that conventional medicine is just as unproven (and far more expensive and dangerous) than the alternatives that are being criticized. For those of us who believe in finding a better way, all we can do is continue to evaluate the research as honestly and objectively as possible, and to use the knowledge we have gained as a means of enhancing the health of the individual, the nation, and the planet.

CONCLUSION AND RECOMMENDATIONS

Although there are still some holes in the boron story, the existing evidence suggests that ingesting adequate amounts of fruits and vegetables and supplementing the diet with 1 to 3 mg/day of boron is a reasonable step to take as an insurance policy against osteoporosis. In addition to providing boron, fruits and vegetables are high in vitamin C, folic acid, vitamin K, and magnesium, all of which help maintain healthy bones. Further, there is evidence these foods in the diet reduce the risk of cancer, heart disease, and some of the other diseases of modern civilization.

Ingestion of nuts in moderation is also recommended. Although nuts tend to be high in fat, they are also a good source of nutritionally important essential fatty acids. It is important that you store nuts in an airtight package, because they contain unsaturated fatty acids which are unstable in the presence of oxygen. If you leave nuts out in the open air, the unsaturated fatty acids will become oxidized to lipid-peroxides, which can cause many harmful effects in the body.

Even if your diet contains these high-boron foods, it may be worthwhile for you to take a broad-spectrum nutritional supplement that contains 1 to 3 mg/day of boron. There is little risk in doing that, and some extra boron in the diet may ultimately prove beneficial, even for people who eat fruits, vegetables, and nuts. Whether or not larger doses should be used will be a topic for future research.

NOTES

1. Pfeiffer, C. C., and E. H. Jenney. 1950. The pharmacology of boric acid and boron compounds. *Bull Natl Formulary Cmte* 18:57–80.

2. Ibid.

3. Nielsen, F. H. 1990. Studies on the relationship between boron and magnesium which possibly affects the formation and maintenance of bones. *Magnesium Trace Elem* 9:61–69.

4. Nielsen, F. H. 1988. Boron—an overlooked element of potential nutritional importance. *Nutr Today* (Jan./Feb.):4–7.

5. Nielsen, F. H. 1989. Effect of boron depletion and repletion on calcium and copper status indices in humans fed a magnesium-low diet. *FASEB J* 3:A760.

6. Follingstad, A. H. 1978. Estriol, the forgotten estrogen? *JAMA* 239:29–30.

7. Lemon, H. M., et al. 1966. Reduced estriol excretion in patients with breast cancer prior to endocrine therapy. *JAMA* 196:1128–1136.

8. Lemon, H. M. 1980. Pathophysiologic considerations in the treatment of menopausal patients with oestrogens; the role of oestriol in the prevention of mammary carcinoma. *Acta Endocrinol* Suppl 233:17–27.

9. Weir, R. J., Jr., and R. S. Fisher. 1972. Toxicologic studies on borax and boric acid. *Toxicol Appl Pharmacol* 23:351–364.

10. Schlettwein-Gsell, D., and S. Mommsen-Straub. 1973. Übersicht spurenelemente in lebensmitteln. IX. Bor. *Int Z Vitaminforsch* 43:93–109.

11. Anonymous. 1992. What Harvard doctors do. *Nutr Forum,* (Jan./Feb.):8.

8

Vitamin B6

Forty years ago, vitamin B6 was considered somewhat of a "second class" vitamin. Whereas other vitamins had been associated with severe deficiency diseases, such as beri beri, pellagra, scurvy, and rickets, there was little evidence that vitamin B6 deficiency was a problem for humans. However, during the past twenty years, numerous studies have demonstrated this vitamin plays a far greater role in health and disease than had been previously thought. There is now evidence that vitamin B6 is of value in the prevention or treatment of asthma, childhood hyperactivity, carpal tunnel syndrome, kidney stones, premenstrual syndrome, heart disease, bladder cancer, and other common problems.

While studying nutrition in the early 1980s, I wondered how a vitamin that had always been of so little use to doctors and nutritionists could suddenly start to look like the next "wonder drug." Were the researchers of yesteryear so unaware that they could have failed to recognize all of these potential applications for vitamin B6? That does not seem to be a likely explanation for the unexpected emergence of vitamin B6. On the contrary, previous generations of scientists had a reputation for being shrewd observers and having keen minds. They knew of many nutritional treatments that are only now being rediscovered. For example, the use of vitamin C for the common cold, popularized by Nobel Laureate Linus Pauling, Ph.D., in the 1970s, had already been mentioned as early as 1944 in an editorial in the *Lancet*. Selenium, which is now being investigated as a possible anticancer nutrient, was used as far back as 1912 to treat cancer patients. Exciting "new" research showing that essential fatty acids improve eczema is not new at all—doctors discovered that in 1933.

A NEW EPIDEMIC OF VITAMIN B6 DEFICIENCY?

It is difficult to believe that a generation of well trained and highly qualified nutritional scientists could have missed so many therapeutic benefits of a well-known vitamin. I believe there is another reason that vitamin B6 has recently become so useful: widespread deficiency of this vitamin is a new problem. That proposition is not as farfetched as it might sound. It is possible that human beings, affected by the stresses of a world becoming increasingly polluted, need a lot more vitamin B6 than we did in the past.

There are two reasons to believe that this may be the case. First, many of the conditions reported to respond to vitamin B6 are either new diseases or are much more prevalent than they used to be. For instance, childhood hyperactivity (also called attention deficit disorder) was hardly mentioned in pediatric journals prior to 1950. Today, on the other hand, hyperactivity is one of the most common problems affecting children. Similarly, carpal tunnel syndrome (a nerve disorder causing numbness, tingling, and weakness in the hands), was relatively unknown 40 years ago, but is a common condition today. Kidney stones have always been around, but there were twice as many per capita in the 1980s as in the 1960s. Premenstrual syndrome (PMS) was also given little attention in the early medical literature, whereas recent studies indicate as many as 70 to 90% of women experience problems with PMS.

What has happened in the past few decades that could have

created an epidemic of vitamin B6 deficiency? It is unlikely that we are dealing strictly with a dietary problem. Although the typical American diet contains less than the Recommended Dietary Allowance (RDA) for vitamin B6, we do not appear to be ingesting any less of this vitamin today than we were fifty years ago. Furthermore, the problem with vitamin B6 seems to be more than just a shortage in the diet. Whereas the RDA for vitamin B6 is only 2 mg/day, the dosages required to treat the conditions mentioned here are often much larger—anywhere from five to several hundred times the RDA. We could not possibly obtain that amount of vitamin B6 from food alone, even from the most well-balanced, nutrient-rich diet imaginable. So, it is not that we are getting less vitamin B6 than before; rather, many of us seem to need a lot more than our grandparents did.

VITAMIN B6 ANTAGONISTS IN THE ENVIRONMENT

The second reason to believe that our need for vitamin B6 has increased is that our environment has been flooded during the past several decades with chemicals that are known vitamin B6 antimetabolites. Any substance that interferes with the metabolism or functioning of a nutrient is called an *antimetabolite* or antagonist. An antimetabolite of vitamin B6 might act in any one of several different ways: It might prevent vitamin B6 from being absorbed, inhibit its passage from the blood to the cells, cause rapid breakdown or excretion of the vitamin, or inhibit its normal biochemical functions. If any of these inhibitory effects are occurring, we would need more vitamin B6 to counteract them.

A widely used group of chemicals called *hydrazines* and *hydrazides* appears to be a major threat to our vitamin B6 metabolism. These chemicals are used extensively in industry as antitarnish agents, as plating materials, and in metal manufacturing. Hydrazines and hydrazides contain a pair of nitrogen molecules bound to each other and are structurally similar to vitamin B_6. A compound whose structure resembles a particular vitamin will often interfere with the function of that vitamin. Other vitamin B6 antagonists are generated by modern food processing. At least one widely used food coloring, several herbicides, and some plant-growth regulators contaminate our food and are also suspected vitamin B6 antimetabolites.[1]

A group of Italian scientists studied how various chemicals affect vitamin B6 metabolism. They found that all compounds with a free hydrazine group strongly inhibited certain biochemical reactions that depend on vitamin B6.[2,3] In another study, various hydrazine compounds injected into mice caused convulsions and death. However, supplementation with vitamin B6 completely prevented the toxicity of four out of five hydrazines and partially prevented toxicity in the other. This study suggested that the adverse effects of vitamin B6 antagonists can be at least partially overcome by providing more of the vitamin.[4]

The proliferation of vitamin B6 antagonists in the environment may explain why doses of this vitamin that exceed RDA levels are usually necessary to treat vitamin B6-responsive disorders. In the case of carpal tunnel syndrome, the usual effective dose is 50 mg/day for a minimum of 6 to 12 weeks. Women with premenstrual syndrome often find that 50 to 200 mg/day of vitamin B6 are required to relieve their symptoms. Children with attention deficit disorder (hyperactivity) who respond to vitamin B6 often need as much as several hundred mg/day. Asthmatics also seem to benefit from doses of vitamin B6 in the range of 50 to 100 mg/day or more.

VITAMIN B6 AND ARTHRITIS

There is also a particular type of arthritis that seems to respond well to vitamin B6. Unlike rheumatoid or osteoarthritis, this type of arthritis has no special name. Vitamin B6-responsive arthritis resembles most closely what used to be called "rheumatism," a term rarely used today. John M. Ellis, M.D., a family physician from Mount Pleasant, Texas, first recognized the pattern of symptoms that respond to vitamin B6.[5] The syndrome described by Ellis included swelling, numbness, tingling, reduced sense of touch in the fingers and hands, and pain in the finger joints which impaired finger movements and weakened the grip. In more severe cases, patients suffered pain and stiffness in the shoulders and sometimes in the elbows and knees, as well. Some also experienced swelling and/or pain in the knees, the muscles between the shoulders and elbows, or the arms and chest. Muscle spasms also occurred in the back of the legs and in the arches of the feet. In some cases, locking of the finger joints and restlessness of the legs would occur. Dr. Ellis found that this entire group of symptoms would usually respond to 50 mg/ day of vitamin B6, as long as they were not due to injury and were associated with at least some of the other symptoms mentioned (isolated symptoms such as a swollen knee or a painful shoulder usually did not respond).

VITAMIN B6, MENOPAUSE, AND HOMOCYSTEINE

Dr. Ellis found vitamin B6 to be most effective in middle-aged women with Heberdon's nodes and arthritis of the interphalangeal joints (the middle group of knuckles), a syndrome known as "menopausal arthritis." This observation suggests that, in addition to any problem with vitamin B6 metabolism created by environmental pollution, the onset of menopause might place further demands on our vitamin B6 needs. This situation appears to be similar to that for folic acid. As discussed in Chapter 6, a potentially harmful compound, homocysteine, builds up in women around the time of menopause. However, supplementing with folic acid reduces the accumulation of this compound. Evidence suggests that a buildup of homocysteine in the body after menopause is one of the factors that promotes accelerated osteoporosis. It is therefore noteworthy that vitamin B6 also plays a role in homocysteine metabolism.

Vitamin B6 supplementation has been shown to reverse the elevated homocysteine levels in some individuals with the genetic condition homocystinuria.[6] In addition, pigs that were fed a diet deficient in vitamin B6 had a fourfold elevation in plasma homocysteine levels.[7] Several other studies have shown that supplementation with vitamin B6, either alone or in combination with other nutrients, lowered plasma homocysteine concentrations in people with initially elevated levels.

If homocysteine is one of the factors that contributes to osteoporosis, then adequate intake of vitamin B6 might help prevent bone loss. However, there are additional ways in which vitamin B6 may promote bone health. This vitamin is a cofactor for the enzyme lysyl oxidase, which crosslinks proteins and connective tissue. Adequate vitamin B6 is therefore required to provide tensile strength and structure to collagen and other structural proteins in bone tissue.

VITAMIN B6 AND OSTEOPOROSIS

Several studies suggest that vitamin B6 is involved in osteoporosis prevention. For example, in rats fed a diet deficient in vitamin B6 and subjected to a fracture of the metatarsal bone, the fractures took longer to heal.[8] In another study, mice fed a vitamin B6-deficient diet had impaired growth of cartilage and defective bone formation.[9] In a separate investigation, rats fed a diet deficient in vitamin B6 developed osteoporosis.[10] In a recent study from England, serum concentrations of pyridoxal-5'-phosphate (the biologically active form of vitamin B6) were below normal in half of twenty patients hospitalized because of a fractured hip.[11] In these patients, the hip fractures had resulted from only minimal trauma, suggesting that severe osteoporosis was an underlying factor. The authors of the study suggested that vitamin B6 deficiency may be one of the causes of hip fractures. However, their study did not rule out the possibility that vitamin B6 levels had declined in response to the trauma of the fracture. To test that possibility, they would have to measure vitamin B6 levels in the same patients a number of months later, after the fracture was healed.

Vitamin B6 and Progesterone

As mentioned, vitamin B6 may prevent osteoporosis either by improving homocysteine metabolism or by enhancing the production of structural proteins in bone. Vitamin B6 may also influence the production of the bone-building hormone progesterone. As discussed in Chapter 15, progesterone plays a crucial role in osteoporosis prevention. There also appears to be a relationship between vitamin B6 and progesterone. In a study performed more than forty years ago, pregnant rats were unable to complete their pregnancies if they were fed a diet deficient in vitamin B6. However, when these vitamin B6-deficient rats were given injections of estrogen and progesterone, most of their pregnancies proceeded normally. Estrogen injections alone were not enough to save the pregnancies; progesterone was essential.[12] This study suggests that vitamin B6 enhances the production or the effectiveness of progesterone. To the extent that progesterone is important for bone health, adequate intake of vitamin B6 is also essential.

THE NEED FOR SUPPLEMENTS

To summarize, evidence suggests that contamination of our environment with vitamin B6 antagonists has resulted in an increase in our requirement for this vitamin. Failure to obtain adequate amounts of this vitamin in the diet may be one of the factors contributing to the increased incidence of osteoporosis in the past three decades.

The need for supplemental vitamin B6 is even more pressing, considering that the typical American diet does not even provide the RDA for this vitamin. In a dietary survey of 127 adolescent females, approximately half of them consumed less than two-thirds of the RDA for vitamin B6. Biochemical measurements suggested vitamin B6 deficiency in 31% of these girls.[13] In another study of adolescent females, marginal or deficient vitamin B6 status was found in 40 to 58% of cases, depending on the method of assessment.[14]

Vitamin B6 deficiency becomes more common with advancing age. According to one report, laboratory evidence of vitamin B6 deficiency was found in 71% of elderly males, 86% of elderly females, 11% of young males, and 30% of young females.[15] Since the elderly are the most susceptible to osteoporosis, the importance of assuring adequate vitamin B6 status during the later years cannot be overemphasized.

Foods high in vitamin B6 include whole grains, watermelon, bananas, fish, chicken, beef, tomatoes, and some nuts. Consumption of excess protein appears to increase the requirement for vitamin B6,[16] which is consistent with the observation that high-protein diets also promote osteoporosis. A significant proportion of the vitamin B6 is lost in the refining of grains, and some losses also occur with cooking, canning, and freezing foods. Cigarette smoking is also associated with vitamin B6 deficiency,[17] possibly because of the presence of hydrazine compounds in cigarette smoke. It is possible that the association between cigarette smoking and osteoporosis is related in part to tobacco-induced vitamin B6 deficiency.

The evidence presented here suggests that, even if one consumes a nutrient-rich diet and does not smoke cigarettes, supplemental vitamin B6 may still be necessary to promote good health.

HOW SAFE IS VITAMIN B6?

The Schaumburg Study

Concerns have been raised about potential toxicity from taking large doses of vitamin B6. In 1983, Herbert Schaumburg, M.D., and colleagues published a report in the *New England Journal of Medicine* titled "Sensory Neuropathy from Pyridoxine Abuse."[18] These doctors presented seven patients in whom severe impairment of sensory nerve function occurred while they were taking between 2,000 and 6,000 mg of vitamin B6 per day. The symptoms typically began with numbness in the feet and instability while walking. This was followed by numbness around the mouth and hands and clumsiness in handling things. In a few cases, nerve biopsies revealed axonal degeneration of the nerve cells. Schaumburg and associates did extensive evaluations on these patients, but were unable to find a cause for this syndrome other than vitamin B6 toxicity. After discontinuing vitamin B6 supplementation, all seven patients had gradual improvement, although some still had neurological abnormalities, even after two or three years.

Some doctors have questioned the validity of Schaumburg's study because there was no clear proof that vitamin B6 had caused the neurologic problems. However, since massive doses of vitamin B6 have been shown to cause similar neurologic damage in animals, the potential for vitamin B6 toxicity in humans should be taken seriously. Other investigators have reported a similar sensory neuropathy in people taking as little as 500 mg/day of vitamin B6. It is important to remember, however, that doses that high are hardly ever necessary.

Furthermore, when nutrients that support the function of vitamin B6 (such as magnesium, zinc, vitamin B-complex, and essential fatty acids) are given simultaneously, less vitamin B6 may be necessary to achieve the desired result. As Roger Williams, Ph.D., pointed out many years ago, nutrients work in the body as a team; a small dose of a wide range of nutrients often works as well as or better than a large dose of a single vitamin or mineral. A number of psychiatrists who use megavitamin therapy say that they rarely, if ever, see vitamin B6-induced neuropathy, even though they often prescribe vitamin B6 in doses far above 500 mg/day. It is the belief of some of these physicians that simultaneous use of many nutrients reduces the risk of vitamin B6 toxicity.

The Dalton Study

One report out of England suggested that vitamin B6 can cause neurological side effects at doses considerably lower than those reported by Schaumburg. Katharina Dalton, M.D., evaluated 103 women attending a premenstrual syndrome (PMS) clinic whose serum vitamin B6 levels were above normal. Sixty percent of these women complained of neurologic symptoms, including paresthesias (unusual sensations in the soft tissue), bone pain, muscle weakness, and numbness. The average dose of vitamin B6 ingested by these women was 117 mg/day for an average duration of 2.9 years. Six months after stopping the vitamin, the symptoms had disappeared in all cases.[19] This study has been used to support the contention of critics that even small doses of vitamin B6 are dangerous.

However, Dalton's study has several serious flaws. In the first place, there was no clear evidence that taking vitamin B6 had anything to do with the neurologic symptoms the women complained of. These symptoms are not uncommon in women with PMS, regardless of whether or not they are taking vitamins. Such symptoms are also seen frequently in people with reactive hypoglycemia and food allergies, both of which overlap with PMS. While the women in this study stopped their vitamin B6 supplements, they also presumably did a number of other things recommended by the PMS clinic, including changing their diet, increasing their exercise, and taking progesterone. The improvement in their symptoms may have had nothing to do with the fact that the women stopped taking vitamin B6.

Thus, the report by Dalton on the alleged toxicity of low doses of vitamin B6 should not be taken as seriously as the work of Schaumburg. Nevertheless, I do see an occasional patient who remarks that taking vitamin B6 makes her feel "weird" or "spacy" or gives her insomnia. These side effects may occur even at small doses, such as 50 mg/day. Children taking vitamin B6 sometimes begin wetting their bed or become irritable and more sensitive to sound. According to Bernard Rimland, Ph.D., these are the symptoms of mild magnesium deficiency.[20] Since vitamin B6 and magnesium work together in the body, taking extra vitamin B6 may increase the need for magnesium. These side effects of vitamin B6 can usually be prevented by taking additional magnesium.

HOW MUCH VITAMIN B6 SHOULD YOU TAKE?

The optimal intake of vitamin B6 is not known and probably varies from person to person, depending on both genetic and environmental factors. As a reasonable approximation, I estimate that most healthy individuals would do well to ingest at least 5 to 25 mg/day of vitamin B6, an amount considerably more than the RDA of 2 mg/day. Individuals with specific vitamin B6-responsive conditions, such as asthma, carpal tunnel syndrome, or premenstrual syndrome often need larger doses for adequate symptom relief. In my experience, doses of 50 to 200 mg/day are nearly always adequate, if vitamin B6 is going to work at all. An occasional patient does seem to need larger amounts, sometimes as high as 1,000 mg/day or more. Some individuals have an apparent defect in their ability to convert pyridoxine (the form of vitamin B6 found in most vitamin pills) into pyridoxal-5'-phosphate (PLP, the biologically active form of the vitamin). In these cases, supplementation with PLP, rather than pyridoxine, may be more effective clinically. However, as PLP is not well absorbed from the intestinal tract, it is not the preferred supplement for individuals who have normal vitamin B6 metabolism.

So, how much vitamin B6 should you take as part of your "insurance policy" against osteoporosis? As mentioned, the data currently available suggest that 25 mg/day would be adequate for most individuals, but taking 50 mg/day is not likely to cause any harm, and this level might turn out to be closer to the optimal intake. Many B-complex vitamin tablets contain 50 to 100 mg of vitamin B6. I recommend that anyone wishing to take more than 100 mg/day of vitamin B6 first consult with a health practitioner who is knowledgeable about nutrition.

NOTES

1. Gaby, A. *The doctor's guide to vitamin B6.* 1984. Emmaus, Pa.: Rodale Press, Chapter 1.

2. Buffoni, F., G. Ignesti, and R. Pirisino. 1977. 3-Hydrazinopyridazine derivatives as inhibitors of the copper containing amine oxidases. *Farmaco* 32:404–413.

3. Buffoni, F., et al. 1980. 3-Hydrazinopyridazine derivatives as inhibitors of pyridoxal-phosphate dependent enzymes. *Farmaco* 35:848–855.

4. Toth, B., and J. Erickson. 1977. Reversal of the toxicity of hydrazine analogues by pyridoxine hydrochloride. *Toxicology* 7:31–37.

5. Ellis, J. M., and J. Presley. 1973. *Vitamin B6: The doctor's report.* New York: Harper & Row, 39–73.

6. Barber, G. W., and G. L. Spaeth. 1967. Pyridoxine therapy in homocystinuria. *Lancet* 1:337.

7. Smolin, L. A., et al. 1983. Homocyst(e)ine accumulation in pigs fed diets deficient in vitamin B6: Relationship to atherosclerosis. *J Nutr* 113:2122–2133.

8. Dodds, R. A., et al. 1986. Abnormalities in fracture healing induced by vitamin B6-deficiency in rats. *Bone* 7:489–495.

9. Silberberg, R., and B. M. Levy. 1948. Skeletal growth in pyridoxine deficient mice. *Proc Soc Exp Biol Med* 67:259–263.

10. Benke, P. J., H. L. Fleshood, and H. C. Pitot. 1972. Osteoporotic bone disease in the pyridoxine-deficient rat. *Biochem Med* 6:526–535.

11. Reynolds, T. M., P. D. Marshall, and A. M. Brain. 1992. Hip fracture patients may be vitamin B6 deficient. Controlled study of serum pyridoxal-5'-phosphate. *Acta Orthop Scand* 63:635–638.

12. Nelson, M. M., W. R. Lyons, and H. M. Evans. 1951. Maintenance of pregnancy in pyridoxine-deficient rats when injected with estrone and progesterone. *Endocrinology* 48:726–732.

13. Kirksey, A., et al. 1978. Vitamin B6 nutritional status of a group of female adolescents. *Am J Clin Nutr* 31:946–954.

14. Ibid.

15. Guilland, J. C., et al. 1984. Evaluation of pyridoxine intake and pyridoxine status among aged institutionalized people. *Int J Vitam Nutr Res* 54:185–193.

16. Levy, B. M. 1950. The effect of pyridoxine deficiency on the jaws of mice. A. Periodontal structures. B. Mandibular condyle. *J Dent Res* 29:349–357.

17. Roepke, J. B., and A. Kirksey. 1983. Effect of smoking and vitamin B6 supplementation during pregnancy on maternal vitamin B6 status and infant birth weight. *Fed Proc* 42:1066.

18. Schaumburg, H., et al. 1983. Sensory neuropathy from pyridoxine abuse: A new megavitamin syndrome. *N Engl J Med* 309:445–448.

19. Dalton, K., M. J. T. Dalton. 1987. Characteristics of pyridoxine overdose neuropathy syndrome. *Acta Neurol Scand* 76:8–11.

20. Rimland, B. 1974. An orthomolecular study of psychotic children. *J Orthomolec Psychiatry* 3(4):371–377.

9

Zinc

Zinc is an important nutrient which participates in more than twenty different biochemical reactions in the body. Zinc is necessary for the activity of insulin, for synthesis of protein and DNA, for wound healing, for taste, smell, and sight, and for normal immune system function. Because of its many functions, zinc deficiency can cause a wide array of effects, including growth retardation, dermatitis, impaired sexual and reproductive function, low resistance to infection, poor wound healing, anemia, and night blindness.

There is evidence that zinc deficiency is relatively common in Americans. In one dietary survey, 68% of adults were receiving less than two-thirds of the Recommended Dietary Allowance (RDA) for zinc in their diet.[1] Widespread dietary zinc deficiency has also been reported in other studies.[2] Refining of sugar and flour, which causes substantial losses of zinc, may be one reason that so many individuals fail to obtain the RDA for this nutrient.

THERAPEUTIC USES OF ZINC

Zinc has been used successfully as a therapeutic agent for a number of different purposes, including acne, rheumatoid arthritis, benign prostatic hypertrophy (prostate enlargement), gastric ulcers, and poor wound healing.

Acne

In one study, thirty-seven individuals with moderate or severe facial acne received either zinc supplements or a tetracyclinelike antibiotic, in a randomized, double-blind trial. After twelve weeks the average improvement in each group was about 70%. Thus, according to this study, zinc is about as effective as tetracycline, one of the standard treatments for acne.[3] Although several other studies have confirmed the effectiveness of zinc in treating acne, a few have yielded negative results. In general, the studies that failed to find zinc effective were of eight weeks' duration or less, apparently not long enough for the therapeutic effect of zinc to become manifest.

Rheumatoid Arthritis

Zinc has also shown promise in treating rheumatoid arthritis. Twenty-four patients with mild to moderate rheumatoid arthritis who had failed to respond to conventional treatments were given either zinc sulfate (220 mg, three times a day; equivalent to about 50 mg of elemental zinc, three times a day) or a placebo, in a twelve-week, double-blind trial. Patients receiving zinc fared better than those receiving placebo in terms of joint swelling, morning stiffness, walking time, and the patients' subjective impression of disease activity.[4] The effectiveness of zinc is apparently due to its mild antiinflammatory action. However, in another study of patients with more severe rheumatoid arthritis, zinc supplements were without benefit.

Prostate Enlargement

Benign prostatic hypertrophy (BPH), a common condition in elderly men which causes various urinary difficulties, also appears to respond to zinc supplements. In one study, 19 men with BPH took 150 mg of zinc sulfate daily for two months, and then 50 to 100 mg daily. In 14 of the 19 cases, the prostate gland became smaller, as determined by rectal examination, X ray, and endoscopy. In an additional 200 men with chronic nonbacterial prostatitis, zinc treatment (50 to 150 mg/day for 2 to 16 weeks) relieved symptoms in 70% of the cases.[5]

Gastric Ulcers

The treatment of gastric ulcers is another area where zinc has been shown to be helpful. Fifteen patients with gastric ulcers received either zinc (50 mg, three times a day) or a placebo, in a three-week double-blind trial. The reduction in the size of the ulcer was about three times as great in the zinc group as in the placebo group. Zinc therapy also produced substantial pain relief in some patients within four days.[6]

Visual Impairment

Individuals with macular degeneration, a common condition in which a portion of the retina deteriorates, resulting in visual impairment or even blindness, have been helped with zinc. In a double-blind trial, 159 patients with macular degeneration were given 45 mg/day of zinc or a placebo. After 12 to 24 months, some patients in the zinc group had further visual deterioration. However, patients receiving zinc had significantly less visual loss than those receiving placebo.[7]

Common Cold

Zinc in the form of lozenges dissolved in the mouth may have value in the treatment of the common cold. In one study, sixty-five individuals suffering from a cold dissolved a 23 mg zinc lozenge or a matching placebo lozenge in their mouths every two hours while awake. After seven days, 86% of the people receiving zinc were free of symptoms, compared to only 46% of those receiving placebo. Side effects of the zinc lozenges were usually minor and consisted mainly of a bad taste and mouth irritation. Zinc lozenges shortened the average duration of a cold by about seven days.[8]

ZINC AND OSTEOPOROSIS

With its multiple effects in the body, it should not be surprising that zinc also plays a role in maintaining bone health. Studies with rats have provided evidence that zinc is essential for normal bone formation.[9] Zinc further enhances the biochemical actions of vitamin D, which is itself involved in calcium absorption and osteoporosis prevention.[10] Because of its essential role in DNA and protein synthesis, zinc is required for the formation of osteoblasts and osteoclasts, as well as for the synthesis of various proteins found in bone tissue. Zinc levels were found low in the serum and bone of elderly individuals with osteoporosis.[11] Low serum zinc levels were also found in people with accelerated bone loss of the alveolar ridge of the mandible (the bone that supports the lower teeth).[12]

Thus, the evidence suggests that zinc deficiency is a relatively common occurrence and that this deficiency may be one factor contributing to the development of osteoporosis. Elderly individuals are probably at increased risk for zinc deficiency because both their food intake and their capacity to absorb nutrients diminish with advancing age. In one study, zinc intake was below the RDA in more than 90% of a group of elderly individuals, ages 60 to 89. A number of these people had both low plasma zinc levels and evidence of impaired immune function, which may have been a result of zinc deficiency.[13]

HOW MUCH ZINC SHOULD YOU TAKE?

Foods rich in zinc include whole grains, meat, chicken, poultry, and legumes. However, even high-nutrient diets often fail to meet the RDA for zinc (15 mg/day). Supplementing with this important mineral may therefore be desirable in many cases. Zinc is available in a number of different forms. It appears that the most efficiently absorbed types of zinc are zinc picolinate, zinc citrate, and chelated zinc. Zinc sulfate does not seem to be as well absorbed as the other forms and also tends to cause gastric irritation. A few supplements contain zinc oxide. This form of zinc is used primarily in medicine for application onto the skin. It is poorly soluble and not well absorbed orally, and is therefore not a preferred source of zinc for oral use.

Most multiple-vitamin and mineral supplements provide 15 to 30 mg/day of zinc. Individual zinc tablets usually contain 15 to 50 mg. Although some short-term studies (three months or less) employed zinc at doses up to 150 mg/day, continued ingestion of such large doses could cause toxicity. Heart rhythm disturbances, abnormalities of cholesterol metabolism, and impairments of immune function have been associated with excessive zinc intake. These side effects are all manifestations of copper deficiency and probably resulted from zinc-induced depletion of copper. Since zinc interferes with the absorption or utilization of copper and, since the typical American diet is often low in copper, it may be unwise to take large doses of zinc without also taking some copper.

For long-term supplementation, I usually recommend 15 to 30 mg/day of zinc. That should probably be balanced with 2 mg/day of copper. For the treatment of certain medical conditions, larger doses of zinc may be advisable for one to three months, after which the dose should be reduced. It is not clear whether high doses of zinc must be balanced with greater amounts of copper. However, when patients are taking 100 mg/day or more of zinc, I usually advise them to take 4 mg/day of supplemental copper. Both zinc and copper will sometimes cause nausea or produce an unpleasant metallic taste in the mouth. These side effects can usually be prevented by reducing the dose.

NOTES

1. Holden, J. M., W. R. Wolf, and W. Mertz. 1979. Zinc and copper in self-selected diets. *J Am Diet Assoc* 75:23–28.

2. Patterson, K. Y., et al. 1984. Zinc, copper, and manganese intake and balance for adults consuming self-selected diets. *Am J Clin Nutr* 40:1397–1403.

3. Michaelsson, G., L. Juhlin, and K. Ljunghall. 1977. A double blind study of the effect of zinc and oxytetracycline in acne vulgaris. *Br J Dermatol* 97:561–566.

4. Simkin, P. A. 1976. Oral zinc sulfate in rheumatoid arthritis. *Lancet* 2:539–542.

5. Bush, I. M., et al. 1974. Zinc and the prostate. Presented at the annual meeting of the American Medical Association, Chicago.

6. Frommer, D. J. 1975. The healing of gastric ulcers by zinc sulphate. *Med J Aust* 2:793–796.

7. Newsome, D. A., et al. 1988. Oral zinc in macular degeneration. *Arch Ophthalmol* 106:192–198.

8. Eby, G. A., D. R. Davis, and W. W. Halcomb. 1984. Reduction in duration of common colds by zinc gluconate lozenges in a double-blind study. *Antimicrob Agents Chemother* 25:20–24.

9. Calhoun, N. R., J. C. Smith, Jr., and K. L. Becker. 1975. The effects of zinc on ectopic bone formation. *Oral Surg* 39:698–706.

10. Yamaguchi, M., and T. Sakashita. 1986. Enhancement of vitamin D3 effect on bone metabolism in weanling rats orally administered zinc sulphate. *Acta Endocrinol* 111:285–288.

11. Atik, O. S. 1983. Zinc and senile osteoporosis. *J Am Geriatr Soc* 31:790–791.

12. Frithiof, L., et al. 1980. The relationship between marginal bone loss and serum zinc levels. *Acta Med Scand* 207:67–70.

13. Bogden, J. D., et al. 1987. Zinc and immunocompetence in the elderly: Baseline data on zinc nutriture and immunity in unsupplemented subjects. *Am J Clin Nutr* 46:101–109.

10

Strontium

Strontium, element number 38 of the periodic table, was discovered in 1808 and was named after Strontian, a town in Scotland. One of the most abundant elements on earth, strontium composes about 0.04% of the earth's entire crust. At a concentration of 400 parts per million, there is more strontium in the earth's crust than carbon. Strontium is also the most abundant trace element in sea water, present at a concentration of 8.1 parts per million. As it is widespread in the environment, living beings have evolved in its presence and have incorporated it into their tissues. The human body contains about 320 mg of strontium, nearly all of which is in bone and connective tissue.

Strontium appears in the periodic table in row IIa, just below calcium. Like calcium, strontium is an element with two positive charges in its ionic form. Because of their chemical similarities, strontium can replace calcium to some extent in various biochemical processes in the body. Specifically, strontium is capable of replacing a small proportion of the calcium in hydroxyapatite crystals of calcified tissues, such as bones and teeth. The presence of strontium in these crystals appears to impart additional strength to these tissues, making them more resistant to resorption. Strontium also appears to draw extra calcium into bones. When rats or guinea pigs were fed increased amounts of strontium, their bones and teeth became thicker and stronger.

STRONTIUM AND DENTAL CAVITIES

The susceptibility of humans to dental cavities may be influenced by the amount of strontium in the diet. In one ten-year study, the United States Navy Dental Service examined the teeth of about 270,000 naval recruits. Of those, only 360 were found to be completely free of cavities. Curiously, 10% of those 360 individuals came from a small area around Rossburg, Ohio, where the water contains unusually high concentrations of strontium. Epidemiologic studies have shown that strontium concentrations of 6 to 10 milligrams per liter in the water supply are associated with a reduced incidence of cavities. Administering these levels of strontium also reduced the incidence of cavities in animal studies.

STRONTIUM AND OSTEOPOROSIS

Strontium has an affinity for bone tissue, tending to migrate to sites in bone where active remodeling is taking place. This behavior suggests that strontium may play a role in bone remodeling. In a study in mice, administering 0.27% strontium in the drinking water increased the rate of bone formation and decreased the rate of bone resorption.[1] In another study, rats given extra strontium had increased bone formation and greater bone density than rats fed a control diet with normal amounts of strontium. These reports suggest that the amount of strontium we ingest may influence our risk of developing osteoporosis, and that strontium may even have a role in the overall management of this condition.

That possibility is supported by the results of several clinical studies. In 1959, researchers at the Mayo Clinic investigated the effect of strontium therapy in thirty-two individuals suffering from osteoporosis.[2] Each patient received 1.7 g of strontium daily in the form of strontium lactate. Some of the patients took strontium for as little as three months, while others continued for as long as three years. The results of strontium therapy were very encouraging. Eighty-four percent of the patients reported marked relief of bone pain, and the remaining 16% experienced moderate improvement. No significant side effects were seen, even with prolonged administration of strontium at levels hundreds of times greater than those found in a typical diet.

Because bone pain is a subjective symptom, and because there was no control group in this study, the possibility of a placebo effect cannot be ruled out. However, it is generally accepted that the placebo effect, that purely psychological benefit, which results from an individual's belief in the treatment or in the doctor, rarely lasts longer than three months. Since some patients maintained their improvement for three full years, it is likely that their improvement was real, rather than psychological.

X rays taken before and after strontium therapy showed a possible increase in bone mass in 78% of the cases, consistent with the symptomatic improvement reported by the patients. Unfortunately, measurement of bone mass in 1959 was rather crude and inexact; more sophisticated tests such as dual photon absorptiometry and CT scanning were not yet available. Nevertheless, the results of this study suggested that strontium deserves consideration as a weapon in the battle against osteoporosis, particularly in view of its wide margin of safety.

STRONTIUM FALLS OUT OF FAVOR

Despite the encouraging results of the Mayo Clinic study, little interest was generated in strontium therapy. As a result, virtually no one attempted to follow up on the initial research. One possible explanation for the lack of interest in strontium is that it is inexpensive and cannot be patented—not exactly the kind of product for which the profit-oriented pharmaceutical industry is willing to fund research. However, it is more likely that strontium fell out of favor because it became confused with strontium-90, a highly dangerous, radioactive component of nuclear fallout, which was being produced during atmospheric testing of nuclear weapons. As a result of this above-ground nuclear testing, radioactive strontium spread throughout the environment and contaminated dairy products and other foods. Because of its affinity for developing and remodeling bone, radioactive strontium accumulated in the bones of both children and adults. The media made us well aware that our bones had become radioactive and that we might develop cancer or some other horrible disease as a result. So, in the minds of many, strontium was poison, plain and simple.

Whatever the reason, the Mayo Clinic study was not followed up for many years. Had doctors and scientists done their homework, however, they would have known that stable (nonradioactive) strontium is virtually nontoxic, even when administered in large doses for prolonged periods of time.

Furthermore, had they studied the history of strontium, they would have learned it had been safely used as a medicinal substance for more than one hundred years. Strontium was first listed in *Squire's Companion to the British Pharmacopoiea* in 1884. Subsequently, strontium was used therapeutically in the United States and Europe. As late as 1955, strontium compounds were still listed in the *Dispensary of the United States of America*. Strontium salts were administered in dosages of 200 to 400 mg/day for decades during the first half of the twentieth century, without toxic effects.

Apparently doctors also failed to consider the possibility that radioactive strontium could be gradually eliminated from the body by repeatedly administering stable strontium. The stable form would slowly replace the radioactive form in bone tissue and radioactive strontium would be excreted in the urine.

NEW RESEARCH

One researcher who never lost interest in strontium was Stanley C. Skoryna, M.D., Ph.D., of McGill University in Montreal. Despite the radioactive strontium scare in the 1950s, Dr. Skoryna continued to investigate the importance of stable strontium in animals. Finally, in 1985, he completed a small-scale study that pointed to a potential role for strontium in the treatment of humans.[3] Three men and three women with osteoporosis were each given 600 to 700 mg/day of strontium in the form of strontium carbonate. Bone biopsies were taken in each patient at the iliac crest (a bone in the lower back just above the hip), both before and after six months of treatment with strontium. Biopsy samples showed a 172% increase in the rate of bone formation after strontium therapy without any change in bone resorption. The patients receiving strontium remarked that the pains in their bones had diminished and their ability to move around had improved. No side effects were reported. However, when strontium therapy was discontinued, symptoms returned in some patients after several months. It was Dr. Skoryna's impression that the response to strontium therapy was better in younger individuals than in older ones.

TREATMENT OF METASTATIC BONE CANCER

Skoryna also tested the effect of strontium on the bone lesions caused by metastatic cancer (cancer that has spread to other tissues). A group of patients with breast cancer or prostate cancer that had spread to the bone was studied.[4] Metastatic bone cancer is usually a tragic condition. The primary cancer has already broken free from its original site and has begun to attack the bones. As the cancer cells multiply out of control, they gradually eat away at the bone tissue. In addition to causing severe pain, metastatic bone cancer can make bones so weak that they break after only minimal trauma, or simply collapse under the body's weight. Deforming and disabling fractures may culminate in loss of mobility and intolerable pain. Metastatic cancer is difficult to treat and usually becomes progressively worse, although successful treatment of the cancer will occasionally cause the bone lesions to regress.

Against the backdrop of this rather dim prognosis, these patients received strontium (in the form of strontium gluconate) for at least three months. The dosage of strontium in this study was 183 to 274 mg/day, an amount somewhat lower than the 600 to 700 mg/day used in the osteoporosis study. However, since strontium gluconate is absorbed more efficiently than strontium carbonate, less strontium was needed to achieve the same blood level. In many cases, the results were clearcut and dramatic. X rays taken before and after strontium therapy demonstrated new mineral deposits in areas of bone that had been eroded by the cancer. In one patient, a vertebra that appeared to be on the verge of collapse showed extensive remineralization. Although much of this newly deposited mineral was no doubt made up of calcium crystals, the presence of strontium was clearly evident by its characteristic appearance on the X rays. These strontium deposits were still visible on X rays taken several months after strontium therapy had been discontinued. Many of the cancer patients reported subjective improvements and gained weight while receiving strontium. No side effects were seen in patients who took up to 400 milligrams of strontium daily, even after a number of years.

These studies indicate that strontium may have a significant role in the prevention and treatment of osteoporosis and other bone diseases, particularly metastatic bone cancer. Because of its lack of toxicity and its low cost, strontium deserves more consideration by doctors and researchers than it has received. Additional research in the area of metastatic bone cancer is urgently needed, as this condition has serious and life-threatening consequences and because current treatments are frequently unsuccessful.

THE FUTURE OF STRONTIUM THERAPY

A number of questions remain unanswered about strontium. For example, what are the optimal doses for osteoporosis and for bone cancer? The daily intake of strontium from food and water is usually on the order of several milligrams per day, far below the range of about 200 to 1,700 mg/day used in clinical trials. Are these very large doses necessary to produce benefits in osteoporosis, or might people see results from supplementing at doses within the nutritional range (say, 2 to 10 mg/day)? Or, would it be best to begin treatment with large doses, and then to give smaller amounts for maintenance?

Does strontium promote the formation of bones that are strong, resilient, and resistant to fracture or does it, like fluoride, produce bones that are thicker, but of relatively poor quality? In the case of metastatic bone cancer, does strontium therapy slow the spread of the cancer? Does it increase the survival time of the patient?

Clearly, these questions cannot be answered without additional research. It should be noted that fluoride is a known poison at relatively low concentrations, whereas strontium is nontoxic, even at much higher concentrations. It is curious, therefore, that so many studies have focused on the effect of fluoride on osteoporosis, while the role of strontium has been largely ignored. Although there are not yet enough data to support the routine use of large doses of strontium for osteoporosis, this type of treatment may be appropriate for some individuals with metastatic bone cancer.

SOURCES OF STRONTIUM

The amount of strontium you ingest each day depends on where your food was grown and on what type of water you drink. Foods grown on soil with a low-strontium content contain less of this mineral than foods grown on high-strontium soil. The strontium content of food varies by twofold or more across the United States.

Water is also a significant source of strontium intake. Since the concentration of strontium in water supplies varies by more than twentyfold in different areas of the country, the amount of strontium in your diet will depend in part on where you live. The strontium content of drinking water varies from less than 1 mg/l to more than 20 mg/l. Therefore, the usual daily intake of strontium can range from as little as 1 mg to more than 10 mg. Addition of strontium to multiple-vitamin and mineral formulas at low doses (0.5 to 3 mg/day) seems like a reasonable thing to do.

NOTES

1. Marie, P. J., and M. Hott. 1986. Short-term effects of fluoride and strontium on bone formation and resorption in the mouse. *Metabolism* 35:547–551.

2. McCaslin, F. E., Jr., and J. M. Janes. 1959. The effect of strontium lactate in the treatment of osteoporosis. *Proc Staff Meetings Mayo Clin* 34:329–334.

3. Marie, P. J., et al. 1985. Histomorphometry of bone changes in stable strontium therapy. In *Trace substances in environmental health XIX,* edited by D. D. Hemphill, 193–208. 3–6 June, University of Missouri, Columbia, Missouri.

4. Skoryna, S. C. 1981. Effects of oral supplementation with stable strontium. *Can Med Assoc J* 125:703–712.

11

Other Nutrients: Copper, Silicon, Vitamin C, Vitamin D

COPPER

Copper performs several different functions in the body: It aids in the production of hemoglobin; is a cofactor in energy metabolism; plays a role in the formation of connective tissue; and has antiinflammatory activity.

A deficiency of copper can cause anemia, a low white blood cell count, impaired immune function, cardiac arrhythmias, and elevated serum cholesterol. Animals fed a copper-deficient diet had elevations of serum uric acid and blood sugar, electrocardiographic abnormalities, and damage to the heart muscle. Elevated blood sugar has also been reported in both humans and animals receiving diets low in copper.

Copper compounds have been found to be effective for treating arthritis.[1,2] In addition, copper supplements may help prevent the development of aortic aneurysm, a serious and sometimes life-threatening condition.[3,4]

Copper and Osteoporosis

Chronic copper deficiency may be a cause of osteoporosis. Rats that were fed a copper-deficient diet had reduced bone mineral content and reduced bone strength.[5,6] Copper supplementation also inhibited bone resorption in test tube studies.[7] Severe copper deficiency is also known to produce abnormalities of bone in growing children. These studies suggest that, in the long term, a diet lacking enough copper might be one of the factors contributing to the development of osteoporosis.

Foods rich in copper include whole grains, nuts, organ meats, eggs, poultry, legumes, and green leafy vegetables. Supplementing the diet with 1 to 2 mg/day of copper may be beneficial and is unlikely to cause any harm. Because zinc interferes with the absorption or utilization of copper, individuals taking large amounts of zinc should also take several milligrams of copper daily to prevent the development of copper deficiency.

Copper Deficiency and Excess

Dr. Carl Pfeiffer, a pioneer in the nutritional treatment of psychiatric illness, pointed out that copper toxicity can cause various psychiatric problems. As a result, many nutrition-oriented practitioners have viewed copper more as a toxic compound than as an essential nutrient. However, while copper overload may, indeed, exist in a small proportion of the population, copper deficiency is probably much more common. In a dietary survey of twenty-two men and women, 81% consumed less than two-thirds of the Recommended Dietary Allowance for copper.[8] Thus, a large proportion of the population may not be getting enough copper in their diet.

SILICON

About twenty years ago, silicon was found to be an essential nutrient. Chicks that were fed a silicon-deficient diet had significantly retarded growth and development. However, when the diet was supplemented with silicon, the growth rate increased by 50% and development returned to normal.[9] Further studies revealed that silicon plays a role in forming cartilage and other connective tissue.

Silicon has also been shown to play a key role in bone health. High concentrations of silicon are found at the calcification sites in growing bone. It has been postulated, therefore, that silicon is involved in an early stage of calcification of bone.[10] Animals that were fed a silicon-deficient diet developed gross abnormalities of the skull, including narrowing of the frontal area and stunting of the parietal, occipital, and temporal bones. X rays and histologic studies revealed reduced numbers of trabeculae (a type of crossfiber that occurs in bone) and inhibited calcification. Analysis of the frontal bones revealed reduced collagen content, indicating that the skull abnormalities were due to impaired production of soft-tissue components of the bone.[11]

It is not known whether the typical American diet provides adequate amounts of silicon. As with other nutrients, subtle deficiencies could result from overconsumption of refined foods. Patients with osteoporosis may require more silicon. One of the best sources of silicon is rice polish or rice bran. Brown rice, which contains the bran portion, also provides a large amount of silicon. This trace mineral is found in some multiple-vitamin and mineral supplements. An herbal product called horsetail is also a rich source of silicon and is sold in health food stores.

VITAMIN C

Ever since Linus Pauling, Ph.D., alerted us in the early 1970s to the importance of vitamin C for the common cold, this vitamin has been the subject of intense research and debate. With the exception of multiple vitamins, vitamin C is the supplement taken most often by Americans. There are a number of good reasons why. Research done over the past several decades has demonstrated many important effects of vitamin C. For instance, there is now reasonably good evidence that vitamin C can help prevent heart disease and cancer, as well as reduce complications resulting from diabetes. In addition, vitamin C has been shown to have a number of important beneficial effects on immune function. Vitamin C also functions as a natural antibiotic. At a concentration of about 10 g/l, vitamin C can kill E. coli, the bacterium most commonly implicated in urinary tract infections. That action may explain why taking 1,000 mg of vitamin C every hour, as recommended by the late Adele Davis, would sometimes clear up urinary tract infections. In addition, studies in the test tube have shown that vitamin C at high enough concentrations is capable of killing virtually every virus known. Based on that observation, some nutrition-oriented physicians have used massive intravenous doses of vitamin C to treat acute hepatitis, infectious mononucleosis, and other viral diseases. In my experience and that of other physicians, massive doses of vitamin C help these viral illnesses to resolve much faster than normal.

Concerns have been raised about the potential toxicity of vitamin C. Specifically, some doctors believe that taking large amounts of this vitamin (such as 4 g/day or more) might increase the risk of developing calcium oxalate kidney stones. However, that concern seems to be unfounded. Abram Hoffer, M.D., a pioneer in the use of megavitamins for schizophrenia, has been using massive doses of vitamin C for more than thirty years and has found no evidence that it causes kidney stones. In my experience, people taking large doses of this vitamin actually seem to have a lower incidence of kidney stones than others. That may be due to the fact that vitamin C binds calcium in the urine, thereby making the calcium less available for stone formation.

Vitamin C and Osteoporosis

Animal studies have shown that vitamin C deficiency can cause osteoporosis.[12] Guinea pigs fed a vitamin C–deficient diet had reduced bone formation and increased bone resorption.[13] Human scurvy, a condition caused by severe vitamin C deficiency, is also associated with various abnormalities of bone. One of the actions of vitamin C on bone is to promote the formation and crosslinking of some of the structural proteins found in bone.

The amount of vitamin C required to prevent osteoporosis is probably relatively small, certainly less than the megadoses being used for other purposes. However, we cannot be sure that elderly individuals are receiving enough of this vitamin in their diet, even if their intake exceeds the RDA. In one study, biochemical evidence of vitamin C deficiency was found in 20% of a group of elderly women, even though they were consuming more than the RDA of 60 mg/day.[14] Although the reason for this finding was not clear, some elderly individuals appeared to need more than 100 mg/day of vitamin C to prevent a deficiency.

A reasonable supplemental dose of vitamin C for the average person is 500 mg/day. Some individuals may wish to take larger amounts, as there is evidence that larger doses may provide added protection against some of the degenerative diseases of modern civilization. In general, vitamin C is quite safe, despite numerous uncritical reports claiming it can be toxic. Excessive intake of vitamin C does cause diarrhea or intestinal upset; these may be lessened by taking the vitamin with food or in a buffered form. Large doses of vitamin C may also interfere with the anticoagulant drug coumadin. Vitamin C may be dangerous in people with severe kidney failure; if you have chronic renal failure, you should probably not take more than 100 mg/day of this vitamin.

VITAMIN D

Vitamin D is required for calcium to be absorbed and deposited into bone tissue. Deficiency of vitamin D in children causes an abnormality of the bones known as rickets. Vitamin D deficiency in adults causes *osteomalacia,* a term that means "soft bones."

Exposing the skin to ultraviolet rays from the sun causes cholesterol within the skin to be converted into vitamin D. Individuals who are out in the sun for reasonable periods of time are therefore unlikely to become deficient in vitamin D. However, those who stay indoors most of the time must obtain their vitamin D from food. The main source of vitamin D is vitamin D–fortified dairy products, fish, eggs, and liver. Vegetarians who do not go outside much are at risk for developing vitamin D deficiency. Certain anticonvulsant drugs can also deplete vitamin D.

The elderly are at increased risk for vitamin D deficiency. Individuals with osteoporosis have been shown to have lower levels of vitamin D than people of similar age without osteoporosis. It is likely, therefore, that vitamin D deficiency is one of the factors that promotes osteoporosis in the elderly.

Supplementation with 200 to 400 units/day of vitamin D as part of a multiple-vitamin and mineral program may be worthwhile. This level of intake is unlikely to pose any risk of toxicity. Prolonged ingestion of large doses of vitamin D, however, can cause toxic effects. Anyone wishing to take more than 400 units/day of vitamin D should consult with a physician.

A hormonal form of vitamin D, known as 1,25-dihydroxyvitamin D3, is being tested as a possible treatment for osteoporosis. Some studies have produced positive results. However, this treatment can occasionally cause dangerous elevations in serum calcium and must be monitored closely.

NOTES

1. Sorenson, J. R. J. 1976. Copper chelates as possible active forms of the antiarthritic agents. *J Medicinal Chem* 19:135–148.
2. Sorenson, J. R. J., and W. Hangarter. 1977. Treatment of rheumatoid and degenerative diseases with copper complexes. A review with emphasis on copper-salicylate. *Inflammation* 2:217–238.
3. Tilson, M. D., and G. Davis. 1983. Deficiencies of copper and a compound with ion-exchange characteristics of pyridinoline in skin from patients with abdominal aortic aneurysms. *Surgery* 94:134–141.
4. Tilson, M. D. 1982. Decreased hepatic copper levels: A possible chemical marker for the pathogenesis of aortic aneurysms in man. *Arch Surg* 117:1212–1213.
5. Follis, R. H., Jr., et al. 1955. Studies on copper metabolism. XVIII. Skeletal changes associated with copper deficiency in swine. *Bull Johns Hopkins Hosp* 97:405–409.
6. Smith, R. T., et al. 1985. Mechanical properties of bone from copper deficient rats fed starch or fructose. *Fed Proc* 44:541.

7. Wilson, T., J. M. Katz, and D. H. Gray. 1981. Inhibition of active bone resorption by copper. *Calcif Tissue Int* 33:35–39.

8. Holden, J. M., W. R. Wolf, and W. Mertz. 1979. Zinc and copper in self-selected diets. *J Am Diet Assoc* 75:23–28.

9. Carlisle, E. M. 1972. Silicon: An essential element for the chick. *Science* 178:619–621.

10. Carlisle, E. M. 1969. Silicon localization and calcification in developing bone. *Fed Proc* 28:374.

11. Anonymous. 1980. Silicon and bone formation. *Nutr Rev* 38:194–195.

12. Hyams, D. E., and E. J. Ross. 1963. Scurvy, megaloblastic anaemia and osteoporosis. *Br J Clin Pract* 17:332–340.

13. Wapnick, A. A., et al. 1971. The effect of siderosis and ascorbic acid depletion on bone metabolism with special reference to osteoporosis in the Bantu. *Br J Nutr* 25:367–376.

14. Morgan, A. F., H. L. Gillum, and R. I. Williams. 1955. Nutritional status of aging. III. Serum ascorbic acid and intake. *J Nutr* 55:431–448.

12

Calcium: Important, But Not the Whole Story

I have placed this discussion of calcium last among the chapters about vitamins and essential minerals, not because calcium is unimportant, but to emphasize one of the main points in this book: that calcium is just one of many nutrients involved in the prevention and treatment of osteoporosis. Furthermore, taking calcium supplements alone, particularly in large amounts, may not do much good and, in some cases, could even cause harm. For years, both the medical profession and the public have focused almost exclusively on calcium as *the* nutrient for building bones. After all, as the argument goes, bones contain a lot of calcium; so if we just take more calcium, our bones will be stronger.

Unfortunately, things are not that simple. The reality is that bone tissue is complex, dynamic, and alive and, like other tissues in the body, has a wide range of nutritional needs. That diversity of nutrient requirements is best illustrated by two studies, one published in 1981, the other in 1990. In the first study, a nutritional supplement containing calcium plus "all known micronutrients" increased the bone density of healthy women two to three times more effectively than did calcium alone.[1] In the second study, a comprehensive program that included diet, hormones, and a broad spectrum of vitamins and minerals produced an astounding 11% increase in the bone mineral content of postmenopausal women in less than one year. Neither calcium alone, nor calcium plus hormones, has ever come close to producing an improvement that great in so short a period of time.[2] These studies are discussed in more detail in Chapters 1 and 5, respectively.

While calcium deficiency is unquestionably one cause of osteoporosis, and while calcium supplementation has preventive or therapeutic value in certain circumstances, we cannot just drink more milk or take more calcium supplements and expect our bones to turn out perfectly fine. But at the same time, ingesting an adequate quantity of absorbable calcium is one of the goals of an osteoporosis prevention program.

Studies on the relationship between calcium intake and osteoporosis are many and varied, and have produced conflicting and confusing results. The consensus of opinion about calcium has changed several times over the years, from effective, to ineffective, to partially effective.

STUDIES ON OSTEOPOROSIS

An earlier study, published in 1964, demonstrated that the intestinal absorption of calcium supplements was markedly lower in people with osteoporosis than in healthy people.[3] Increasing the calcium intake of osteoporotic individuals would, in theory, compensate for this reduced absorption, thereby improving bone mass. It would be a number of years before the technology would be available to measure small changes in bone mass. However, when that technology did become available, the first thing many investigators looked at was calcium.

Calcium and Bone Mass

In a 1977 study, seventy-two postmenopausal women were given either calcium supplements (800 mg/day), estrogen, or no treatment. Untreated women continued to lose bone, while those given estrogen did not. Bone loss in the calcium-treated group was intermediate.[4] In another study several years later, twenty elderly women were given 2.25 ounces of cheese per day and a daily supplement containing 350 mg of calcium, 270 mg of phosphorus, and 399 units of vitamin D. After six months, the average bone density had increased significantly. Eleven women had an increase in bone density, three had no change, and six had decreased bone density at the end of the study.[5]

Other reports have also shown that calcium improves bone mass. In one such report, calcium supplements reduced the number of vertebral crush fractures in women with postmenopausal osteoporosis by about 50%. Whereas untreated women were suffering an average of nearly one collapsed vertebra every year, calcium treatment reduced this figure by half. When calcium and estrogen were given together, the incidence of vertebral fractures fell by 82%.[6] In a more recent study, 169 women, ages 35 to 65, received 1,500 mg/day of calcium or a placebo for four years. The calcium group lost less bone mineral than did the placebo group. The results of calcium supplementation were more pronounced in postmenopausal than in premenopausal women.[7] Another study of a group of 76 healthy postmenopausal women investigated the relationship between dietary calcium intake and osteoporosis. Bone mineral density of the lumbar spine was measured at the time the dietary survey was taken and was then repeated seven months later. Women whose daily calcium intake was less than 405 mg lost bone at a significantly greater rate than did those whose calcium intake was greater than 777 mg/day.[8]

However, a number of other studies have shown that calcium has little or no value in the prevention or treatment of osteoporosis. In a study by B. Lawrence Riggs, M.D., of the Mayo Clinic, 106 healthy women, ages 23 to 84 years, were observed for periods of 2.6 to 6.6 years. During that time, there was no correlation between dietary calcium intake (which ranged from 260 to 2,035 mg/day) and the rate of bone loss.[9] In another study, women in the early postmenopausal period who received 2,000 mg/day of supplemental calcium had approximately the same rate of bone loss as those given a placebo.[10] Other research has shown that, in people with osteoporosis, a high calcium intake has no effect either on bone formation or bone resorption.[11]

These conflicting results are consistent with the viewpoint that calcium deficiency is only one of many causes of osteoporosis and that not everyone who has osteoporosis is actually deficient in calcium. In one study, the prevalence of skeletal calcium deficiency was assessed in fifty-six osteoporotic patients, using a combination of three measurements: (1) total mineral content per gram of bone, (2) bone density, and (3) sodium/calcium ratio in bone. The results of these measurements suggested that only 25% of the patients had a skeletal calcium deficiency, even though all of them had osteoporosis. Supplementation with calcium and vitamin D for two years corrected the skeletal calcium deficiency in all cases but did not improve bone mass in the 75% of osteoporotic individuals who had initially normal skeletal calcium levels.[12]

Calcium and Teeth

Calcium has been found to prevent resorption of the alveolar bone, the bone structure that supports the teeth. Forty-six individuals being fitted for dentures were given either a daily supplement containing 750 mg of calcium and 375 units of vitamin D or a placebo, in a one-year, double-blind study. The average amount of alveolar bone loss in the supplemented group was 36% less than that in the placebo group.[13] If calcium can prevent or delay alveolar bone loss, then it may allow people to retain their natural teeth, thereby reducing the need for dentures.

In summary, calcium deficiency is only one of a number of factors related to osteoporosis risk. Calcium supplementation may be of value for preventing not only bone loss, but hypertension, high cholesterol, and colon cancer, as well (see Chapter 13). Calcium should not be taken alone, but as part of a comprehensive nutritional program.

HOW MUCH CALCIUM DO YOU NEED?

For prevention and treatment of osteoporosis, I usually recommend 600 to 1,200 mg/day of supplemental calcium, an amount somewhat lower than that suggested by other doctors. If there is evidence of nutrient malabsorption, the recommended dosage may be higher. I always advise my patients to combine calcium with the other nutrients discussed in this book, such as vitamin K, folic acid, vitamin B6, magnesium, manganese, zinc, copper, boron, silicon, and so on. A number of products on the market provide a good balance of all of these vitamins and minerals. My experience in nutritional medicine has taught me that providing a smaller amount of all required nutrients is usually more effective than using a large dose of a single nutrient.

Many women are advised by their internist or gynecologist to take 1,500 mg/day of calcium. That figure is based on studies which suggest that elderly women need 1,500 mg/day to maintain calcium balance (that is, to avoid losing calcium from their body).[14] However, when doctors focus on that 1,500 mg/day figure, they often forget to include calcium obtained from the diet. The average dietary intake of calcium by elderly women is about 500 mg/day, whereas that of younger women is usually higher; around 600 to 1,000 mg/day. If a woman is taking 1,500 mg/day of supplemental calcium, then her total calcium intake will be in the range of 2,000 to 2,500 mg/day—more than what is needed to maintain calcium balance.

CAN TOO MUCH CALCIUM DEPLETE OTHER MINERALS?

Although there is no proof that taking these larger doses is harmful, there are some concerns about possible adverse consequences of taking too much calcium. Specifically, taking too much calcium might interfere with the absorption or utilization of other essential nutrients. Studies have shown that calcium interferes with the absorption of iron. This inhibition is more pronounced with increasing calcium doses, but can occur even at intakes of calcium commonly found in the diet.[15] Oral administration of excess calcium also decreased the absorption and tissue levels of zinc in rats.[16] Although short-term studies (up to forty-two days) in healthy males failed to find that 2,000 mg/day of calcium affected zinc balance,[17] it is possible that taking high doses of calcium for years could deplete zinc.

Perhaps the most significant concern about taking too much calcium is that it might lead to magnesium deficiency. As discussed in Chapter 5, magnesium deficiency appears to be one of the most widespread and most clinically significant nutritional problems in the United States. Taking excessive amounts of calcium might further compromise what is already, for many individuals, a rather precarious situation with respect to magnesium status. The adverse effect of calcium supplementation on magnesium levels has been demonstrated in animal studies. Rats that were fed a diet containing 1.5% calcium had lower levels of magnesium in various tissues of their body than rats fed only one-third that much calcium.[18]

Magnesium Deficiency Causes
Abnormal Calcium Metabolism

Calcium and magnesium have a number of chemical similarities and interact in many important ways in biochemical systems. For example, magnesium has been shown to prevent the formation of calcium oxalate crystals, the most common cause of kidney stones. In fact, in people who suffer from recurrent stone formation, administering 500 mg/day of magnesium reduced the recurrence rate by as much as 90%.[19] Magnesium also functions as nature's "calcium-channel blocker," preventing the transfer of calcium into places within the cell where it could do harm.[20] In animal studies, magnesium deficiency causes calcium deposits in the kidney, a condition known as nephrocalcinosis. There is also evidence that magnesium deficiency promotes atherosclerosis (hardening of the arteries),[21] which is characterized by, among other things, calcification of arterial tissue. These studies indicate that magnesium deficiency can cause various abnormalities of calcium metabolism, resulting in the formation of calcium deposits in places where calcium does not belong.

This calcium–magnesium interaction presumably extends to bone tissue, as well. As discussed in Chapter 5, osteoporotic women who were deficient in magnesium had abnormal (and presumably more fragile) calcium crystals in their bones, whereas osteoporotic women with normal magnesium status had normal calcium crystals in bone. This effect of magnesium deficiency on bone could be considered yet another example of abnormal calcification, similar to that induced in the urinary tract, kidney, and aorta by magnesium deficiency.

WHY SUCH HIGH DOSES OF CALCIUM?

Doctors who recommend 1,500 mg/day of calcium do so because of a study that showed that such a large dose is necessary for elderly women to maintain calcium balance. However, few doctors who prescribe 1,500 mg/day of supplemental calcium have stopped to consider what maintaining calcium balance actually means. In nutritional studies, the term *balance* refers to the difference between the amount of a nutrient entering the body and the amount leaving. If someone is in positive calcium balance, they are excreting less than they are taking in, and their total-body calcium content is increasing. If they are in negative calcium balance, they are excreting more than they are taking in, and their total-body calcium content is declining. For a person in calcium balance (also called *zero calcium balance*) the intake and output are the same, and the total-body calcium content remains steady. Doctors assume that maintaining calcium balance is the same as preventing bone loss.

Unfortunately, that assumption may not be correct. In an elderly individual with chronic degenerative diseases, the arteries and joints may be slowly calcifying, and additional calcium deposits may be developing in muscle or other soft tissue. That type of calcium retention is not exactly desirable; on the contrary, it is a manifestation of disease progression. So, if someone is losing a little bit of bone while, at the same time, calcifying their soft tissues, their total-body calcium content might remain the same, even though their body is falling apart. There is no way of knowing to what extent this type of scenario actually occurs. What I am concerned about, however, is that taking excessive amounts of calcium without adequate magnesium could accelerate both osteoporosis and soft-tissue calcification. Furthermore, this unhealthy situation might be misinterpreted as desirable, if calcium balance is the sole criterion upon which results are based. It is interesting to note that human autopsy studies have shown a close correlation between osteoporosis and calcification of the abdominal aorta.[22] Since magnesium deficiency can promote both osteoporosis and aortic calcification, it is possible that magnesium is the primary factor and that calcium is secondary.

BALANCE CALCIUM WITH MAGNESIUM

Therefore, if someone chooses to take large doses of calcium, I strongly urge them to increase their magnesium intake, as well. There are many different opinions among nutrition-oriented practitioners concerning the proper ratio of calcium to magnesium. The traditional ratio is 2 mg of calcium for every 1 mg of magnesium. For example, many nutritional supplement programs provide 800 to 1,000 mg of calcium and 400 to 500 mg of magnesium daily. Some doctors, however, are of the opinion that these minerals should be provided in equal amounts. Other practitioners actually recommend a reversal of the ratio: 2 mg of magnesium for every 1 mg of calcium.

Surprisingly, there is virtually no research aimed at determining the optimal calcium/magnesium ratio in the diet. The osteoporosis study by Dr. Abraham, which reported such a dramatic improvement in bone mass (see Chapter 5), did supply more daily magnesium (600 mg) than calcium (500 mg). In practice, I have seen an occasional patient with premenstrual syndrome or other symptoms who clearly responded better to 800 mg of magnesium and 400 mg of calcium than to the reverse ratio. Perhaps our best bet at present is to follow the lead of those who have reported the best results and keep the calcium level low to moderate, while raising the magnesium intake. We just do not know yet what the best approach is. Additional research in this area is urgently needed. One thing we do know is that taking calcium by itself, particularly large amounts, may not do a whole lot of good, and has the potential to cause harm.

NOTES

1. Albanese, A. A., et al. 1981. Effects of calcium and micronutrients on bone loss of pre- and postmenopausal women. Scientific exhibit presented to the American Medical Association, 24–26 January, in Atlanta, Georgia.

2. Abraham, G. E., and H. Grewal. 1990. A total dietary program emphasizing magnesium instead of calcium. Effect on the mineral density of calcaneous bone in postmenopausal women on hormonal therapy. *J Reprod Med* 35:503–507.

3. Spencer, H., et al. 1964. Absorption of calcium in osteoporosis. *Am J Med* 37:223–234.

4. Horsman, A., et al. 1977. Prospective trial of oestrogen and calcium in postmenopausal women. *Br Med J* 2;789–792.

5. Lee, C. J., G. S. Lawler, and G. H. Johnson. 1981. Effects of supplementation of the diets with calcium and calcium-rich foods on bone density of elderly females with osteoporosis. *Am J Clin Nutr* 34:819–823.

6. Riggs, B. L., et al. 1982. Effect of the fluoride/calcium regimen on vertebral fracture occurrence in postmenopausal osteoporosis. *N Engl J Med* 306:446–450.

7. Smith, E. L., et al. 1989. Calcium supplementation and bone loss in middle-aged women. *Am J Clin Nutr* 50:833–842.

8. Dawson-Hughes, B., P. Jacques, and C. Shipp. 1987. Dietary calcium intake and bone loss from the spine in healthy postmenopausal women. *Am J Clin Nutr* 46:685–687.

9. Riggs, B. L., et al. 1987. Dietary calcium intake and rates of bone loss in women. *J Clin Invest* 80:979–982.

10. Riis, B., K. Thomsen, and C. Christiansen. 1987. Does calcium supplementation prevent postmenopausal bone loss? A double-blind, controlled clinical study. *N Engl J Med* 316:173–177.

11. Lafferty, F. W., G. E. Spencer, Jr., and O. H. Pearson. 1964. Effects of androgens, estrogens and high calcium intakes on bone formation and resorption in osteoporosis. *Am J Med* 36:514–527.

12. Burnell, J. M., et al. 1986. The role of skeletal calcium deficiency in postmenopausal osteoporosis. *Calcif Tissue Int* 38:187–192.
13. Wical, K. E., and P. Brussee. 1979. Effects of a calcium and vitamin D supplement on alveolar ridge resorption in immediate denture patients. *J Prosthetic Dent* 41:4–11.
14. Heaney, R. P., et al. 1982. Calcium nutrition and bone health in the elderly. *Am J Clin Nutr* 36:986–1013.
15. Hallberg, L, et al. 1992. Calcium and iron absorption: mechanism of action and nutritional importance. *Eur J Clin Nutr* 46:317–327.
16. Adham, N. F., and M. K. Song. 1980. Effect of calcium and copper on zinc absorption in the rat. *Nutr Metab* 24:281–290.
17. Spencer, H., et al. 1984. Effect of calcium and phosphorus on zinc metabolism in man. *Am J Clin Nutr* 40:1213–1218.
18. Smith, K. T., and K. R. Luhrsen. 1986. Trace mineral interactions during elevated calcium consumption. *Fed Proc* 45:374.
19. Johansson, G., et. al. 1982. Effects of magnesium hydroxide in renal stone disease. *J Am Coll Nutr* 1:179–185.
20. Iseri, L. T., and J. H. French. 1984. Magnesium: Nature's physiologic calcium blocker. *Am Heart J* 108:188–193.
21. Vitale, J. J., et al. 1957. Interrelationships between experimental hypercholesterolemia, magnesium requirement and experimental atherosclerosis. *J Exp Med* 106:757–767.
22. Boukhris, R., and K. L. Becker. 1972. Calcification of the aorta and osteoporosis. *JAMA* 219:1307–1311.

13

How to Take Calcium

As discussed in Chapter 12, while increasing your intake of calcium may help prevent osteoporosis, it should not be taken alone, but, rather, as part of a comprehensive nutritional program.

In addition to its beneficial effect on osteoporosis, there are other reasons to obtain adequate calcium in your diet. Recent studies have shown that extra calcium may also be useful as a treatment for hypertension (high blood pressure), to lower serum cholesterol and triglyceride levels, and possibly to prevent colon cancer.

CALCIUM AND HIGH BLOOD PRESSURE

Several studies have demonstrated a blood pressure–lowering effect of calcium in individuals with hypertension. In one such study, forty-eight patients with hypertension received 1,000 mg/day of calcium or a placebo, each for eight weeks, in a double-blind crossover trial. Compared with the placebo, calcium significantly lowered both systolic and diastolic blood pressure.[1] Although the average blood pressure reductions were small (an average of 3.8 to 5.6 mm of Hg for systolic and 2.3 mm of Hg for diastolic blood pressure), such small changes often represent the difference between needing blood pressure medication and getting by without it. Similar results with calcium therapy have been reported by other researchers.[2]

LOWERING CHOLESTEROL AND TRIGLYCERIDES

Calcium also shows promise as a safe and inexpensive way of reducing cholesterol and triglyceride levels. Ten individuals with hyperlipidemia (elevated blood fats) were given calcium carbonate at a dose of 2 g per day for one year. The average serum cholesterol level fell significantly after six months (from 349 to 278 mg/dl; a 20% reduction) and fell further to 262 mg/dl (a 25% reduction) after one year. The average serum triglyceride level fell by 35% after one year, from 327 to 213 mg/dl.[3]

PREVENTION OF COLON CANCER

Recent studies suggest that calcium may play a role in the prevention of colon cancer. In an epidemiologic study, there was an inverse association between dietary calcium intake and the risk of developing colon cancer. In other words, the more calcium in the diet, the lower the risk of colon cancer. This effect was more pronounced for men than for women.[4] The possible calcium/cancer connection was further supported by observations that calcium supplementation reduced the proliferation of colonic cells, implying a reduction in colon cancer risk.[5]

HEALING GUM DISEASE

One other possible benefit of calcium supplementation is in relation to periodontal (gum) disease. Ten patients with periodontal disease received 1 g/day of calcium for six months. Calcium therapy markedly reduced or eliminated bleeding of the gums, reduced tooth mobility, and improved or eliminated gingivitis (inflammation of the gums). In many cases, the structure of the bones supporting the teeth improved, and new alveolar bone appeared in some instances.[6] Most dentists believe that gingivitis causes damage to the bony structures supporting the teeth and that this damage culminates in tooth loss. But, the authors of the study presented here suggest that the reverse may actually be true: that alveolar bone loss caused by calcium deficiency results in excessive tooth mobility, which, in turn, promotes the development of periodontal disease.

ARE YOU GETTING ENOUGH CALCIUM?

The studies described here and in Chapter 12 underscore the importance of insuring adequate daily calcium intake. The Recommended Dietary Allowance (RDA) for calcium is 800 mg/day for adults and 1,200 mg/day for adolescents, pregnant women, and nursing mothers. Many people fail to achieve these targets for calcium intake.

In one study, the daily intakes of calcium by men and women 65 years or older were 600 and 480 mg, respectively.[7] Elderly individuals may have greater difficulty obtaining enough calcium for several reasons. First, because metabolism slows with age, the total food intake and, therefore, the amount of calcium ingested declines. Second, because of dental problems, older people may be forced to reduce their intake of vegetables, which are relatively high in calcium. Third, some elderly individuals have difficulty getting to the supermarket and, therefore, may not be able to keep dairy products and fresh food in stock. As a result, they may be forced to rely on processed foods, which tend to be lower in calcium.

Adolescents, on the other hand, often have ravenous appetites, but their poor food choices may cause their calcium intake to fall short. Unbalanced diets pose a particular problem for pregnant and lactating women because their calcium requirements are greater. Failure to obtain enough calcium during adolescence and early adulthood will prevent a woman from achieving her maximum potential bone mass during her bone-building years, making her more susceptible to osteoporosis later in life.

ARE DAIRY PRODUCTS DANGEROUS?

The most significant source of calcium in the American diet is, of course, dairy products, which include milk, cream, cheese, cottage cheese, and yogurt. An eight-ounce glass of milk or a cup of yogurt contains about 250 mg of calcium. Most types of cheese provide about 200 mg of calcium per ounce. The easiest way to achieve the RDA for calcium is to include several helpings per day of dairy products in your diet.

Problems with Cow's Milk

However, a number of scientists, doctors, and nutritionists have serious concerns about possible adverse effects of dairy products on human health. It is frequently pointed out that humans are the only beings on earth who consume the milk of another species. The consequences of this unprecedented cross-species experiment can only be imagined. Cow's milk is an extremely complex food, designed to serve the needs of baby cows and bulls, not humans. It contains many different proteins which, because they are foreign to humans, have the potential to cause allergic reactions.

Cow's milk is probably the most common cause of infantile colic. In fact, some infants are so sensitive to cow's milk that they develop colic, even when exclusively breast-fed, if their mother consumes any milk in her diet. In one study, colic was cured in 68% of nineteen breast-fed infants by eliminating milk products from the mother's diet.[8] Intolerance to cow's milk can also cause a serious condition in infants called *necrotizing enterocolitis,* characterized by abdominal distension, bloody diarrhea, perforation of the bowel wall, and even death.[9] A less severe, but far more common problem in early childhood is anemia. Gastrointestinal bleeding due to milk allergy has been shown to be a common cause of anemia in children.[10] Milk allergy is also frequently implicated as a factor in childhood asthma.[11]

Milk Allergies

Another potentially serious disease related to milk allergy is *nephrotic syndrome,* a condition in which the kidneys spill an abnormally large amount of protein into the urine. Individuals with nephrotic syndrome suffer from protein deficiency and severe fluid retention, and may ultimately develop permanent kidney damage. The standard treatment for nephrotic syndrome is corticosteroids (cortisonelike drugs) or other immune system suppressing medications. In one study, allergy to cow's milk was found to be a cause of nephrotic syndrome in five of six children studied. Elimination of milk from their diet resulted in marked improvement.[12]

While most pediatricians believe that children "outgrow" milk allergy, nutrition-oriented practitioners find that milk allergy remains a significant problem for many adults. In my experience and in the experience of many of my colleagues, dairy products rank with wheat as the two most common symptom-evoking foods in allergic adults. The gastrointestinal symptoms associated with irritable bowel syndrome and inflammatory bowel disease (ulcerative colitis and Crohn's disease) can often be traced to milk allergy. In addition, allergy to milk products is frequently found to be a cause of chronic nasal congestion, low-level fatigue and depression, migraine headaches, and arthritic symptoms.

I have even seen some patients in whom the symptoms of multiple sclerosis were clearly related to ingestion of dairy products. If milk allergy was discovered within the first several years of the diagnosis, the symptoms of multiple sclerosis could be controlled completely for years by strict avoidance of dairy products. On the other hand, symptoms would recur rapidly, sometimes within hours, if dairy products were reintroduced into the diet.

Lactose Intolerance

Lactose intolerance is another potential problem for milk drinkers. Even if you are not allergic to dairy products, you may lack the intestinal enzymes necessary to break down the milk sugar lactose. The presence of undigested lactose in the intestinal tract can cause abdominal pain, bloating, gas, and diarrhea. Individuals with lactose intolerance who are not also allergic to the proteins in milk may be able to tolerate milk products if the lactose has been predigested or removed. Most cheeses contain little or no lactose and can therefore be used by lactose intolerant people.

In the production of yogurt, some of the lactose in milk is converted by fermentation to lactic acid. In addition, yogurt itself contains some lactase, the enzyme responsible for digesting lactose. Some of this enzyme can actually become implanted in the human small intestine when yogurt is eaten, thereby improving the capacity of lactose intolerant individuals to digest lactose. Yogurt may, therefore, be an acceptable food for some people with lactose intolerance, as long as they are not also allergic to milk protein.

Regular milk can also be predigested by adding some lactase enzyme to it. Lactase is commercially available, as is predigested milk. Since the lactose in predigested milk is converted to the sugars glucose and galactose, this type of milk has a somewhat sweet taste.

Does Drinking Milk Prevent Osteoporosis?

I estimate that as many as 15 to 20% of the patients I have seen during the past thirteen years are allergic to milk. Many others have lactose intolerance. But what about the majority of individuals who appear to tolerate dairy products without any problems? Should they be consuming a lot of dairy products in the hope of preventing osteoporosis?

To be sure, there are several studies that indicate drinking milk is associated with greater bone mass and a reduced risk of developing osteoporosis. However, in some developing countries where milk is not an important part of the diet and calcium intake is low by Western standards, osteoporosis is actually less common than in the United States. It is difficult to tell whether drinking milk itself prevents osteoporosis, or whether consumption of dairy products is merely associated with other beneficial behaviors.

Americans have been told for years that milk is a wonderful, health-promoting, bone-building food. Many famous superstar athletes have been paid by the dairy industry to deliver that message to the public. Although a number of reputable scientists disagree with the claim that milk is good for us, we have had it well drummed into our heads that "milk does a body good." People who drink milk are, therefore, presumably more interested in their health than are nonmilk drinkers. Health conscious individuals also tend to consume less sweets, caffeine, alcohol, meat, and white bread, do more exercise, and take nutritional supplements. So, it is possible that the greater bone mass in milk drinkers is due to these other factors, rather than to milk per se.

Does Milk Cause Heart Disease?

Even if drinking milk does prevent osteoporosis, there is another reason to question whether it should be a routine part of the human diet. Research by Kurt Oster, M.D., a cardiologist from Bridgeport, Connecticut, has provided strong evidence that cow's milk contains a substance that can damage arteries and promote atherosclerosis (hardening of the arteries).[13] Oster was not as much concerned about the high fat and cholesterol content of whole milk as he was about a specific protein molecule, an enzyme called *xanthine oxidase*. This enzyme, which is involved in the metabolism of DNA, occurs naturally in cow's milk. According to Oster, xanthine oxidase is capable of damaging cell membranes, particularly those of the human arterial wall, by reacting with membrane fatty acids. Normally, this enzymatic reaction would not pose a threat to humans, because a food-derived enzyme such as xanthine oxidase would not survive the digestive process. Enzymes are delicate and complex protein molecules that lose their biologic activity when they are altered or partially degraded. So, after milk is acted upon by stomach and pancreatic juices, xanthine oxidase would no longer be xanthine oxidase, but rather, just a bunch of amino acids.

However, according to Oster's hypothesis, the modern-day process of homogenizing milk changes that scenario. Milk is homogenized to extend shelf life and to prevent the cream from rising to the top. The process of homogenization reduces the size of fat particles in the cream portion of milk and disperses them evenly throughout the milk. Oster's research suggests that homogenization causes protein molecules such as xanthine oxidase to become surrounded by a protective coating of fat molecules. Furthermore, in homogenized milk, the size of fat particles is reduced to the point where they can cross the intestinal tract and enter the bloodstream. As a result, homogenizing milk protects xanthine oxidase from being destroyed by digestive juices and allows it to be absorbed intact into the bloodstream. Once inside the body, the enzyme finds its way to the arteries, where it begins to wreak havoc.

In support of his hypothesis, Oster pointed out that antibodies to bovine (cow) xanthine oxidase have been found in the blood of individuals with atherosclerosis. The presence of these antibodies strongly suggests that xanthine oxidase from cow's milk somehow finds its way into the human body. In addition, xanthine oxidase of bovine origin has been found in human atherosclerotic plaques. While human beings also have a xanthine oxidase enzyme, it does not occur in arterial tissue. Furthermore, the xanthine oxidase identified by Oster in atherosclerotic plaques was shown by immunologic tests to be clearly of bovine origin.

Oster has had many critics and his hypothesis has been generally ignored by conventional medicine. However, Oster's thesis is consistent with epidemiologic studies related to heart disease and dairy product consumption. Whereas the incidence of cardiovascular disease in populations around the world is correlated with consumption of homogenized milk (which is high in xanthine oxidase), no such correlation exists with the intake of butter or cheese (which contain little or no biologically active xanthine oxidase).[14] Furthermore, independent investigators, using radioisotope studies, have demonstrated the entrance of bovine xanthine oxidase into the bloodstream of rabbits from orally administered cow's milk.[15]

Oster's research presents a reasonable case that consuming homogenized milk is one of the causes of atherosclerosis. While no one knows for sure whether this hypothesis is correct, it certainly calls into question dairy industry claims that milk makes us healthy. A food that is frequently allergenic, difficult for a large proportion of the population to digest, and a possible cause of one of the major diseases of Western civilization may not be the ideal choice for a dietary source of calcium.

SHOULD YOU CONSUME DAIRY PRODUCTS?

Based on currently available data (it would be nice to have more), a number of recommendations can be made:

1. Individuals with symptoms suggestive of food allergy should determine the specific foods to which they are allergic (see Chapter 17). Those allergic to dairy products should not use them as a dietary source of calcium. In addition to perpetuating symptoms, repeatedly ingesting allergenic foods may cause gastrointestinal damage, resulting in impaired absorption of calcium and other nutrients.
2. People with lactose intolerance can usually handle cheese and yogurt, which contain little or no lactose. Predigested milk is also usually acceptable.
3. Because of the concerns related to Oster's xanthine oxidase hypothesis, completely avoiding homogenized milk may be advisable, even by those who do not have milk allergy or lactose intolerance. This applies to whole milk, 2% fat milk, and 1% fat milk. Cheese, yogurt, evaporated milk, and butter contain no biologically active xanthine oxidase. These foods may be consumed in moderation.

   Several brands of skim milk have been analyzed for xanthine oxidase activity. One brand had no detectable activity, while another had a substantial amount. Since skim milk is fat-free and does not require homogenization, any xanthine oxidase present in skim milk would probably be destroyed by digestive juices. Therefore, skim milk is probably acceptable.[16] It should be noted, however, that skim milk is not a complete food for infants, who should be given whole milk if they have to be given milk at all.

NONDAIRY SOURCES OF CALCIUM

If you consume several helpings of dairy products each day, you should have no trouble obtaining the RDA for calcium of 800 mg/day. However, if you consume little or no dairy products, then it will be difficult to meet the RDA by diet alone. The best nondairy sources of calcium are dark green leafy vegetables and broccoli. One exception is spinach. Although spinach contains substantial amounts of calcium, most of it is in the form of calcium oxalate, which is poorly absorbed. In one study, healthy volunteers absorbed only 5.1% of the calcum in spinach.[17] Citrus fruits, fish with edible bones (such as mackerel), and legumes are also good sources; and whole grains provide some calcium, as well.

Most individuals who do not consume dairy products should consider taking calcium supplements. In most cases, doses of 400 to 1,200 mg/day are appropriate. The dose should be individualized on the basis of age, diet, and the presence or absence of osteoporosis or other diseases.

IS THERE A DIFFERENCE
BETWEEN CALCIUM SUPPLEMENTS?

There is a great deal of controversy about the optimal form of calcium for supplementation. Many different calcium salts are commercially available, including carbonate, lactate, gluconate, citrate, malate, and microcrystalline hydroxyapatite. However, despite many claims for the superiority of one form of calcium over another, there are surprisingly few studies showing that the type of calcium supplement you take makes much difference.

In one study of healthy volunteers, there was no difference in the way the body utilized calcium from milk, oyster shell, or dolomite, and the carbonate, lactate or gluconate salts of calcium.[18] In another study, healthy men ingested calcium from milk and from five different calcium salts (acetate, lactate, gluconate, carbonate, and citrate). The average amount of calcium absorbed ranged from 27 to 39% and did not differ significantly among any of the calcium sources.[19]

Other research suggests that calcium obtained from calcium citrate, calcium citrate malate, calcium orotate, calcium aspartate, or extracts of whole bone may be preferable to other forms of calcium. However, this research is by no means conclusive. For those of you who are interested in a more detailed discussion of the various calcium salts, please see the addendum to this chapter.

DOES YOUR CALCIUM TABLET DISSOLVE?

In addition to the type of calcium salt, you should also consider the physical form of the supplement. Studies have shown that some calcium tablets are packed together in such a way that they do not dissolve effectively. A home test can be done to determine whether your calcium supplement will dissolve: Place one tablet in six ounces of vinegar at room temperature. Stir every 2 to 3 minutes. After 30 minutes, the tablet should have disintegrated (not dissolved) into fine particles. If it has not disintegrated, it should not be used.[20] In a recent survey, 11 of 21 commercial calcium products failed a similar test, indicating that they are unlikely to be efficiently absorbed.[21] Because of this potential problem with tablet dissolution, capsules or chewable tablets may be the best forms in which to take calcium supplements.

Whatever form of calcium you choose, it is important to remember that no single nutrient functions in the body by itself. Calcium should be part of a comprehensive program that includes all of the nutrients necessary for good health and strong bones.

ADDENDUM: COMPARISON OF DIFFERENT
FORMS OF CALCIUM (TECHNICAL INFORMATION)

One study suggested that the body absorbs calcium citrate more readily than other calcium salts.[22] However, in that study, absorption was estimated from the increase in urinary calcium excretion. Since citrate alone (as opposed to calcium citrate) has been shown to increase urinary calcium excretion,[23] one cannot be certain that this is an appropriate criterion for assessing absorption of calcium citrate. Another study has shown that calcium absorption from a combination of calcium citrate and calcium malate was 36.2%, significantly greater than that from calcium carbonate (26.4%).[24]

Calcium orotate and calcium aspartate have been recommended by Hans Nieper, M.D., a noted German physician and scientist. According to Nieper, these calcium salts are better utilized than other forms of calcium. However, I am unaware of any studies which demonstrate these calcium salts are superior to others.

Calcium from MH

Calcium from microcrystalline hydroxyapatite (MH), an extract of whole bone, was absorbed more efficiently than calcium gluconate in one study.[25] However, in another study, the absorption of calcium from MH was less efficient than that from other sources.[26] MH has received attention because it has been shown to slow bone loss in patients with rheumatoid arthritis who were receiving corticosteroids.[27] However, this study did not compare the effect of MH with that of other calcium supplements.

MH has also been shown to reverse bone loss in patients with a liver disease known as primary biliary cirrhosis.[28] In that study, MH was more effective than calcium gluconate. It could be argued that the presence of phosphorus in MH explains the superior results in patients with primary biliary cirrhosis. This condition is associated with malabsorption and deficiency of both calcium and phosphorus. It is not clear whether MH would be superior to other forms of calcium in situations where phosphorus status is normal. On the other hand, a study done fifty years ago showed that bone meal (which is similar to MH) was more effective in the treatment of children with "growing pains" than was dicalcium phosphate.[29] Thus, there may be additional factors present in bone meal or in MH that would make it a preferred source of calcium.

Lead Contamination

One important consideration for each of these products is possible contamination with lead. Because lead is so widespread in our environment and accumulates in bones, the possibility of lead contamination of bone meal or MH must be kept in mind. If you are interested in using either of these products, make sure that you are dealing with a reputable manufacturer and that the products have been analyzed for lead content. Lead concentrations less than 2 parts per million are acceptable.

NOTES

1. McCarron, D. A., and C. D. Morris. 1985. Blood pressure response to oral calcium in persons with mild to moderate hypertension. *Ann Intern Med* 103:825–831.
2. Resnick, L. M., J. E. Sealey, and J. H. Laragh. 1983. Short and long-term oral calcium alters blood pressure (BP) in essential hypertension. *Fed Proc* 42:300.
3. Bierenbaum, M. L., A. I. Fleischman, and R. I. Raichelson. 1972. Long-term human studies on the lipid effects of oral calcium. *Lipids* 7:202–206. *Note:* The reduction in triglyceride levels was not statistically significant, because of the small sample size. However, a 35% reduction is rather dramatic and should be investigated further.
4. Slattery, M. L., A. W. Sorenson, and M. H. Ford. 1988. Dietary calcium intake as a mitigating factor in colon cancer. *Am J Epidemiol* 128:504–514.
5. Wargovich, M. J., and A. R. Baer. 1989. Basic and clinical investigations of dietary calcium in the prevention of colorectal cancer. *Prev Med* 18:672–679.
6. Krook, L., et al. 1972. Human periodontal disease. Morphology and response to calcium therapy. *Cornell Vet* 62:32–53.
7. Heaney, R. P., et al. 1982. Calcium nutrition and bone health in the elderly. *Am J Clin Nutr* 36:986–1013.
8. Jakobsson, I., and T. Lindberg. 1978. Cow's milk as a cause of infantile colic in breast-fed infants. *Lancet* 2:437–439.
9. de Peyer, E., and J. Walker-Smith. 1977. Cow's milk intolerance presenting as necrotizing enterocolitis. *Helv Paediatr* 32:509–515.
10. Anyon, C. P., and K. G. Clarkson. 1971. Cows' milk: a cause of iron-deficiency anemia in infants. *N Z Med J* 74:24–25.
11. Rowe, A. H., and E. J. Young. 1959. Bronchial asthma due to food allergy alone in ninety-five patients. *JAMA* 169:1158–1162.

12. Sandberg, D. H., et al. 1977. Severe steroid-responsive nephrosis associated with hypersensitivity. *Lancet* 1:388.

13. Oster, K. A. 1976. The treatment of bovine xanthine oxidase initiated atherosclerosis by folic acid. *Clin Res* 24:512A. See also Oster, K. A., D. J. Ross, and H. H. Dawkins Richmond. 1983. *The XO factor,* New York: Park City Press.

14. Oster, Ross, and Dawkins Richmond, 44, 229.

15. Anonymous. 1987. Atherosclerosis. *Am Family Physician* 36(6):250.

16. Oster, Ross, and Dawkins Richmond, 229–233.

17. Heaney, R. P., C. M. Weaver, and R. R. Recker. 1988. Calcium absorbability from spinach. *Am J Clin Nutr* 47:707–709.

18. Kohls, K., C. Kies, and H. M. Fox. 1986. Calcium supplement use by humans; comparison of bioutilization, convenience and cost. *Fed Proc* 45:374.

19. Sheikh, M. S., et al. 1987. Gastrointestinal absorption of calcium from milk and calcium salts. *N Engl J Med* 317:532–536.

20. Kobrin, S. M., et al. 1989. Variable efficacy of calcium carbonate tablets. *Am J Kidney Dis* 14:461–465.

21. Shangraw, R. 1987. Factors to consider in the selection of a calcium supplement. Special Topic Conference on Osteoporosis, October.

22. Nicar, M. J., and C. Y. C. Pak. 1985. Calcium bioavailability from calcium carbonate and calcium citrate. *J Clin Endocrinol Metab* 61:391–393.

23. Gomori, G., and E. Gulyas. 1944. Effect of parenterally administered citrate on the renal excretion of calcium. *Proc Soc Exp Biol Med* 56:226–228.

24. Miller, J. Z., et al. 1988. Calcium absorption from calcium carbonate and a new form of calcium (CCM) in healthy male and female adolescents. *Am J Clin Nutr* 48:1291–1294.

25. Windsor, A. C. M., et al. 1973. The effect of whole-bone extract on [47]Ca absorption in the elderly. *Age Ageing* 2:230–234.

26. Reid, I. R., et al. 1986. The acute biochemical effects of four proprietary calcium preparations. *Aust NZ J Med* 16:193–197.

27. Nilsen, K. H., M. I. V. Jayson, and A. S. J. Dixon. 1978. Microcrystalline calcium hydroxyapatite compound in corticosteroid-treated rheumatoid patients: A controlled study. *Br Med J* 2:1124.

28. Epstein, O., et al. 1982. Vitamin D, hydroxyapatite, and calcium gluconate in treatment of cortical bone thinning in postmenopausal women with primary biliary cirrhosis. *Am J Clin Nutr* 36:426–430.

29. Martin, E. M. 1944. Report on the clinical use of bone meal. *Can Med Assoc J* 50:562–563.

14

Estrogen Replacement Therapy

One of the most difficult decisions faced by women entering menopause is whether or not to take estrogen. Estrogen replacement therapy has obvious benefits, such as relief of hot flashes, depression, and vaginal atrophy. Estrogen has also been clearly shown to slow the rate of postmenopausal bone loss and to reduce the incidence of osteoporotic fractures by about 50%. However, there are also definite risks and side effects associated with taking estrogen. The discussion in this chapter is designed to help you understand the risks and benefits of estrogen replacement therapy, in order to help you make a more informed decision.

The fact that osteoporosis is far more common in women than in men and that bone loss accelerates after menopause suggests that an age-related decline in female sex hormones plays an important role in the development of osteoporosis. This concept is supported by the observation that women whose ovaries have been surgically removed lose bone at an unusually rapid rate for about four to six years following the operation. In women with intact ovaries, the amount of estrogen and other hormones secreted by the ovaries begins to decline around the time of menopause. The adrenal glands compensate in part for this decline in ovarian function by secreting certain androgens (male hormones) into the bloodstream, which are converted elsewhere in the body into estrogens. However, despite this contribution from the adrenal glands, the amount of estrogen in the body falls at menopause.

SYMPTOMS OF MENOPAUSE

Menopause occurs around 50 to 52 years of age. At that time, the reduced estrogen secretion is no longer sufficient to produce menstrual cycles. In most women, during the first several years after menopause the amount of estrogen produced from adrenal sources is sufficient to support normal structure and the function of secondary sex tissues, such as the breasts, urethra, vagina, and vulva. With increasing age, however, as secretion of adrenal estrogen precursors declines these estrogen-dependent tissues begin to atrophy. The progressive reduction in estrogen levels leads first to a loss of ovulation and menstruation, followed by vaginal and vulvar tissue contraction, and finally, atrophy of all estrogen-dependent tissues. This prolonged period of progressive decline in estrogen levels, from age 40 to 70 and beyond, is called the *female climacteric.* The single point at which menstruation ceases is known as menopause.

The most common symptoms associated with menopause are hot flashes, those uncomfortable sensations of intense body heat accompanied by flushing of the skin on the head, neck, and chest and sometimes profuse perspiration. These symptoms may last anywhere from a few seconds to several minutes. In some women they occur only occasionally, while others are plagued with hot flashes several times every hour. For most women, hot flashes last about 1 to 2 years; however, in about 25% of women they may last as long as 5 years. In most cases, treatment with low doses of estrogen successfully relieves these symptoms.

As estrogen deficiency becomes more severe, atrophy of the vaginal mucous membranes may occur, resulting in vaginal itching or inflammation, pain on intercourse, and narrowing of the vaginal opening. Thinning or inflammation of the urethra (the urinary tract opening) may also occur and may cause pain on urination, frequent urination, or a tendency to leakage of urine. Estrogen replacement therapy, either orally or by direct application to the atrophied tissues, is nearly always successful in reversing these symptoms.

ESTROGEN PREVENTS OSTEOPOROSIS

One of the main reasons doctors recommend estrogen replacement therapy is that it prevents osteoporosis. It is now well established that estrogen replacement therapy reduces the incidence of osteoporotic fractures by approximately 50%. Estrogen works by preventing the increase in bone resorption that occurs at menopause. In contrast, estrogen has no effect on bone formation. Thus, estrogen therapy does not reverse established osteoporosis. However, if estrogen therapy is discontinued, bone loss resumes, possibly at an accelerated rate. Therefore, for estrogen therapy to be successful in the prevention of osteoporosis it must be started early, before significant bone loss has occurred, and continued indefinitely.

ESTROGEN, ATHEROSCLEROSIS, AND HEART DISEASE

Estrogen may prevent atherosclerosis (hardening of the arteries). Estrogen therapy raises serum levels of HDL cholesterol, the "good cholesterol," which has been shown to protect against the development of cardiovascular disease. Recently, estrogen has also been shown to prevent the oxidation of cholesterol. An increasing body of research suggests that oxidized cholesterol, not cholesterol itself, is a primary cause of atherosclerosis. If estrogen can prevent the oxidation of cholesterol, it should also protect against the development of atherosclerosis.

Unfortunately, research on the effect of estrogen on heart disease is conflicting. Whereas some studies have shown that estrogen replacement therapy reduces the risk of heart disease by as much as 50 to 70%, other studies have shown a 50% increase in the risk of cardiovascular disease in women taking estrogen.

SIDE EFFECTS OF ESTROGEN

Women taking birth control pills have an increased risk of developing potentially dangerous blood clots, high blood pressure, and blood sugar abnormalities. It is thought that these side effects are due to the estrogen component of the pill. Since the dosage of estrogen in postmenopausal replacement therapy is lower than that found in birth control pills, these side effects have not been found to be a problem for postmenopausal women. However, both estrogen replacement therapy and birth control pills have been shown to increase the risk of gallbladder disease. Estrogen therapy could also conceivably worsen estrogen-dependent conditions such as uterine fibroids and endometriosis. Other side effects of estrogen include breast pain or worsening of fibrocystic breast disease, vaginal bleeding, high blood pressure, nausea, vomiting, headaches, jaundice, fluid retention, and impaired glucose tolerance.

ESTROGEN AND CANCER

Estrogen replacement therapy is known to increase the risk of endometrial (uterine) cancer. Studies show that women taking estrogen are between four and thirteen times more likely to develop cancer of the uterus than women who are not taking estrogen. Fortunately, the increased risk of endometrial cancer attributable to estrogen can be entirely eliminated if estrogen therapy is combined with a progestogen. However, progestogens themselves sometimes cause significant side effects, including dangerous blood clots, fluid retention, breast tenderness, jaundice, nausea, insomnia, and depression. In addition, most women who take a combination of estrogen and progestogen have a return of menstrual bleeding, which may require periodic biopsies of the uterine lining to screen for cancer.

Of greatest concern is the possibility that estrogen therapy could promote the growth of estrogen-sensitive breast cancers. In view of the fact that 1 in 9 women in this country will develop breast cancer, any increase in risk is a serious problem. An estimated 180,000 cases of breast cancer occurred in the United States in 1992, 32% of all female cancers.

At least twenty-eight studies have looked at the relationship between estrogen replacement therapy and breast cancer. These studies have been reviewed by five different teams of investigators, using a statistical technique called meta-analysis. These analyses suggested that estrogen replacement therapy is associated with an increase in the risk of breast cancer, ranging from 1 to 30%.[1] In none of the studies was the increased risk statistically significant; in other words, these differences could have occurred by chance. However, because breast cancer is such a common problem, even a small increase in risk can have profound implications. For example, given a 1 in 9 (11.1%) chance of developing breast cancer, a 30% increase in risk (the highest number reported in the meta-analyses) would increase the overall breast cancer risk to 14.4%. If this worst-case scenario is accurate, then for every 1,000 women receiving estrogen replacement therapy, there would be 33 more cases of breast cancer (above and beyond the 111 already expected).

WHO SHOULD RECEIVE ESTROGEN?

Thus, despite certain clear benefits of estrogen replacement therapy, there is still considerable uncertainty among doctors about who should receive estrogen and for how long. Although the benefits are obvious, so are the risks. An estimated 30% of postmenopausal women do not lose significant amounts of bone. If these women do not have menopausal symptoms, then there is little reason for them to subject themselves to the risks of estrogen therapy. Unfortunately, it is not possible to predict accurately who will develop osteoporosis. However, periodic monitoring of bone mass using dual photon absorptiometry or CT scanning is useful for identifying established osteoporosis or for detecting those women who are losing bone at a rapid rate. Some women have chosen to hold off on taking estrogen until these tests demonstrate the need for it.

TYPES OF ESTROGEN MEDICATION

The most commonly used form of estrogen is known as *conjugated estrogens,* such as Premarin. Conjugated estrogens are not themselves physiologically active, but are converted within the body into active compounds. The physiologically active form of estrogen, 17β-estradiol, is not well absorbed when taken by mouth. The small amount that does get absorbed is largely destroyed by the liver before entering the bloodstream. However, 17β-estradiol is well absorbed through the skin and is the form of estrogen used in the newer estrogen patches. Estrogen patches are preferable to conjugated estrogens because they deliver the natural form of estrogen directly into the bloodstream in a slow, sustained manner. In that respect, estrogen patches resemble natural estrogen secretions more closely than do conjugated estrogens. Application of a single patch maintains a relatively constant serum level of 17β-estradiol for approximately 3.5 days; therefore, the patches must be changed twice a week. The patch has been found to be clinically effective, in terms of relieving menopausal symptoms and maintaining bone density.

Estrogen is also available as a vaginal cream. At one time it was thought that estrogen cream could be used to relieve local symptoms, such as vaginal dryness and atrophy, without being absorbed into the system. However, it is now known that estrogen is well absorbed through the vaginal tissue into the blood and can cause the same side effects as orally administered estrogen.

With the various types of estrogens and the different patterns of dosing, with or without the use of progestogens, there are numerous possible regimens that can be prescribed for estrogen replacement therapy. No single pattern has gained wide acceptance. In fact, in a survey of 283 gynecologists in the Los Angeles area, fully

84 different patterns of estrogen replacement therapy were being employed. The main patterns were

1. cyclic estrogen alone
2. continuous estrogen alone
3. cyclic estrogen plus cyclic progestogen
4. continuous estrogen plus cyclic progestogen
5. continuous estrogen plus continuous progestogen
6. progestogen alone (cyclic or continuous)[2]

REDUCING CANCER RISK WITH ESTRIOL

As mentioned previously, the greatest concern about estrogen therapy is that it might cause cancer. Whether or not this concern is well founded (and we do not yet know, for sure), some women will not take estrogen and some doctors will not prescribe it, because of their fear of promoting cancer. Fortunately, there is a way to take estrogen that does not appear to increase the risk of cancer. In fact, this "alternative" method of estrogen replacement therapy could actually prevent cancer. Sadly, most physicians are unaware that there is another way to administer estrogen that is apparently as effective as, and probably safer than, the standard approach.

When doctors talk about estrogen, they usually forget that estrogen is not a single substance. On the contrary, estrogen exists in the body in at least three forms. The first two forms, *estrone* (abbreviated E1) and *estradiol* (abbreviated E2) are relatively potent estrogens, in terms of their ability to relieve hot flashes and other menopausal symptoms. Unfortunately, E1 and E2 also appear to be the forms of estrogen that promote cancer. The estrogen preparations usually prescribed for women contain E1 and/or E2 or other related compounds that are converted in the body into E1 or E2. However, a third form of estrogen, known as *estriol,* also occurs naturally in the body. And, in contrast to the cancer-promoting effects of the other two estrogenic compounds, estriol has actually been shown to have anticancer activity.

Estriol is considered a weak estrogen because more estriol is required, compared to standard estrogen medications, to relieve menopausal symptoms. However, if an appropriate dose of estriol is given, these symptoms often do improve. A dose of 2 to 4 mg of estriol is considered equivalent to, and as effective as, 0.6 to 1.25 mg of conjugated estrogens or estrone.[3]

Estriol and Endometrial Hyperplasia

The standard estrogen preparations frequently cause a potentially precancerous proliferation of the uterine lining, known as *endometrial hyperplasia*. In contrast, most investigators have found that estriol does not cause endometrial hyperplasia, even when given in doses as high as 8 mg/day. In one study, for example, fifty-two women with severe menopausal symptoms were given estriol continuously for six months in doses of 2 to 8 mg/day. Improvements in symptoms occurred within one month and persisted as long as estriol therapy was continued. The degree of symptom improvement was related to the dose—moderate at 2 mg/day, but marked at a dose of 8 mg/day. Estriol therapy also produced an improvement in vaginal atrophy and in the quality of the cervical mucus. However, endometrial biopsies failed to show hyperplasia in any case, regardless of the dosage of estriol used. Breakthrough bleeding also was not a problem.[4]

These observations suggest that estriol may be an appropriate choice where estrogen therapy is concerned. When judged in terms of endometrial proliferation, one of the unwanted effects of estrogen therapy, estriol is a weak estrogen. By other criteria, however, such as improvement in hot flashes and vaginal atrophy, estriol is a more potent estrogen.[5] Thus, estriol therapy may produce some of the beneficial effects of estrogen therapy, while avoiding the undesirable side effects. In one report, large doses of estriol did cause some proliferation of endometrial tissue. However, the women given estriol in that study were also receiving a progestogen (such as Provera).[6] So far, no one has reported that administration of estriol by itself causes endometrial hyperplasia.

Estriol and Breast Cancer

The other area of major concern with regard to estrogen therapy is in relation to breast cancer. Although the many studies on this issue have yielded no clear proof that estrogen promotes breast cancer, neither could these studies rule out the possibility that estrogen increases cancer risk by as much as 30%. Because that chance exists, safer forms of estrogen therapy are badly needed. Here, again, estriol may be an ideal choice.

More than twenty-five years ago, it was shown that estriol was not only noncarcinogenic, but that it inhibited the breast cancer-promoting effect of estradiol in mice.[7] Estriol also inhibited the development of breast cancer in rats induced by two different chemical carcinogens.[8] Because of this anticancer effect of estriol in animals, Dr. H. M. Lemon investigated whether estriol has any relationship to breast cancer in humans. He developed a mathematical formula, which he called the *estrogen quotient,* a measure of the ratio of the cancer-inhibiting estrogen (estriol) to the cancer promoting estrogens (estrone plus estradiol). If the estrogen quotient was high, that meant there was a large amount of estriol relative to the others and that the risk of cancer would presumably be reduced. Conversely, if the estrogen quotient was low, that meant there was little estriol present, compared to the levels of the cancer-promoting estrogens. Women with a low estrogen quotient would, therefore, be expected to have a higher risk of cancer. Lemon collected twenty-four-hour urine samples from both healthy women and those with breast cancer. He found that the median estrogen quotient in healthy women was 1.3 prior to menopause and 1.2 after menopause. Only 21% of these women had estrogen quotients below normal. In contrast, among twenty-six women with breast cancer who had not received hormonal therapy or recent surgery, the median estrogen quotients were 0.5 and 0.8, respectively, with 62% of the women having values below normal.[9] These results indicate that women with breast cancer have a low level of estriol relative to the other forms of estrogen.

Another study also suggested a relationship between estriol and breast cancer prevention. Seventeen women with fibrocystic breast disease were given vitamin E, 600 units/day, for two months. Women with this condition are thought to have an increased risk of developing breast cancer. Because vitamin E has been reported both to relieve fibrocystic breast disease in humans and to inhibit chemically induced breast cancer in rats,[10] the effect of vitamin E on estriol levels was measured. Vitamin E treatment produced an 18% increase in the ratio of estriol to estradiol.[11] This increase in the relative concentration of estriol after administration of vitamin E may explain in part the reported anticancer effects of this vitamin.

Because of the apparent safety of estriol, doctors began carefully testing it in women with breast cancer that had metastasized (spread to other areas of the body). The dosage of estriol ranged from 2.5 to 15 mg/day. The results of this preliminary study were remarkable: In fully 37% of those receiving estriol, there was either a remission or no further progression of the metastatic lesions. These results were far better than expected, considering the natural history of metastatic breast cancer.[12]

OTHER ADVANTAGES OF ESTRIOL

Estriol has several other possible advantages over the commonly used forms of estrogen. Because estriol produces very little endometrial proliferation, it rarely causes postmenopausal vaginal bleeding. One of the problems with conventional estrogen therapy is that it is sometimes difficult to distinguish normal hormone-induced bleeding from pathologic bleeding (such as that due to cancer). Consequently, many women on hormone replacement therapy are subjected to diagnostic D&Cs (dilatation and curettage) and sometimes even unnecessary hysterectomies. The use of estriol would probably reduce the need for these procedures. Estriol may also more effectively lower the risk of thromboembolism (blood clots in the veins or lungs) than other estrogens.[13]

THE FORGOTTEN ESTROGEN

Despite these encouraging studies with estriol, there has been little interest among physicians in the United States in this "other" estrogen. In contrast, estriol has been available in Europe for many years. In an attempt to educate American doctors about this important substance, Dr. Alvin H. Follingstad, of Albuquerque, New Mexico, published an article in the *Journal of the American Medical Association*, titled, "Estriol, the forgotten estrogen?"[14] Follingstad concluded in that article that estriol should be given to women who need estrogen therapy but who are at high risk for developing cancer. Considering that 1 in 9 women in the United States is expected to develop breast cancer, a case can be made that nearly the entire population is at risk. The role of estriol in postmenopausal hormone replacement therapy should, therefore, be given a closer look.

But, fifteen years after Follingstad alerted American doctors about the "forgotten estrogen," estriol is still ignored by all but a small group of open-minded physicians in this country. Many doctors have never heard of estriol; others refuse to try it for no other reason than the fact that it is different. For many physicians in this country, the code of conformity is very powerful. Living under the constant threat of rejection by colleagues, scrutiny by medical disciplinary boards, malpractice lawsuits, and an unwritten law that they are supposed to know everything, doctors often find it easier to run with the pack than to risk being different—even if being different means practicing a superior brand of medicine.

CLINCIAL USE OF ESTRIOL

Tri-estrogen

Fortunately, some doctors are not intimidated by institutionalized mediocrity. One physician who has been unwilling to relinquish the joy of thinking for himself is Jonathan V. Wright, M.D., of Kent, Washington. For more than fifteen years, Dr. Wright has been internationally recognized as a leading authority in nutritional medicine, although, in the spirit of humility and noncompetitiveness, he prefers to think of himself as a "trailing authority."[15]

In the early 1980s, Dr. Wright began working with estriol as an alternative to the conventional estrogen medications. Eventually, he came to the conclusion that the optimal way to use estriol was not by itself, but in combination with the more commonly used estrogens. The reason was that, in some women, the amount of estriol required to relieve menopausal symptoms was as high as 10 to 15 mg/day. Studies had also suggested that as much as 12 mg/day of estriol was needed to prevent osteoporosis.[16] Unfortunately, some women could not tolerate those relatively large amounts of estriol. In some cases, they caused nausea severe enough to require a dosage reduction.

Dr. Wright therefore developed an estrogen formula designed to maximize the benefits of estrogen, while minimizing the risks. By measuring serum levels and urinary excretion of the three naturally occurring estrogens, he concluded that the most appropriate proportions for a combination pill would be 80% estriol, 10% estrone, and 10% estradiol. Wright named his formula tri-estrogen. He found that 2.5 mg of tri-estrogen is usually effective for relieving menopausal symptoms such as hot flashes and vaginal atrophy, although some women need 5 mg/day. Wright generally administers tri-estrogen in a cyclical fashion, twenty-five days per month, adding natural progesterone for twelve days at the end of the cycle. With the 2.5 mg dose of tri-estrogen and a low dose of progesterone, he hardly ever encounters withdrawal bleeding, although it does sometimes occur if larger doses of tri-estrogen and progesterone are given. According to Wright, the 2.5 mg dose of tri-estrogen is therapeutically equivalent to 0.625 mg of conjugated estrogens (Premarin), whereas the 5 mg dose is equivalent to 1.25 mg of conjugated estrogens.

Osteoporosis Prevention

Although this specific combination of estrogenic hormones has not been tested with respect to osteoporosis prevention, its beneficial effect on menopausal symptoms suggests that it would also be effective for osteoporosis. Tri-estrogen may therefore be an ideal estrogen preparation for women who need estrogen therapy, but in whom the usual forms of estrogen pose an unacceptable risk. In some cases, estriol alone, at doses of 2 to 8 mg/day, is effective for relief of symptoms. However, as mentioned, those doses of estriol may not prevent osteoporosis. The decision about which type of estrogen to use can, therefore, be rather complicated.

The decision is made more difficult when one takes into account the work of John Lee, M.D., described in Chapter 15. According to Lee, natural progesterone alone effectively reverses osteoporosis, and additional estrogen does not make the progesterone more effective. If Lee is correct, then estrogen is necessary only to relieve menopausal symptoms, not for osteoporosis prevention. Thus, in cases where estriol alone relieves symptoms, that would be the preferred treatment. However, if the dose of estriol required to relieve symptoms causes nausea, then tri-estrogen might be preferable.

The appropriate choice of estrogen should be evaluated on an individual basis. At this point, additional research is needed before we will know how best to balance estrogen therapy to maximize osteoporosis prevention, while minimizing cancer risk. However, it is encouraging to know that we have safer options than those currently being offered by the average doctor.

ESTROGENS IN FOOD

In many situations, the use of estrogen is medically inadvisable, while in other cases, a woman may simply choose not to accept the risks of therapy. Occasionally, however, the effects of estrogen can be mimicked by eating specific foods that contain compounds with estrogenic activity. These compounds, which include genistein, daidzein, and equol, are known as *phytoestrogens* (plant-derived estrogens). Soy products such as tofu, miso, aburage, atuage, koridofu, soybeans, and boiled beans contain large amounts of phytoestrogens. High intake of phytoestrogens may partly explain why hot flashes and other menopausal symptoms are so infrequent in

Japanese women.[17] However, it is not known whether phytoestrogens will help prevent osteoporosis. Other foods that have been found to have estrogenic activity include cashew nuts, peanuts, oats, corn, wheat, apples, almonds, and alfalfa.[18,19] Ginseng also has estrogenic activity and some herbalists use it as an alternative to estrogen. Ginseng should be used with caution, however, as an overdose can cause high blood pressure, anxiety, and insomnia.

ADDING TESTOSTERONE

In some cases, adding the male hormone testosterone to an estrogen regimen may be more effective than estrogen alone. The normal ovary manufactures testosterone and continues to do so, even after menopause. However, women who have had their ovaries removed may exhibit signs of testosterone deficiency, including loss of libido and breast tenderness. Women who have undergone natural menopause also occasionally develop testosterone deficiency, which can be diagnosed by measuring the level of testosterone in the blood. Testosterone-deficient women may also find that the usual menopausal symptoms do not respond to estrogen therapy. In these cases, treatment with Estratest, a medication that contains both estrogen and testosterone, may reverse these symptoms. Correction of testosterone deficiency may also have a beneficial effect against osteoporosis. In a two-year study, administration of Estratest markedly increased bone density.[20]

However, Estratest is not for all women. In most cases, the ovary continues to produce adequate amounts of testosterone, even after menopause. The adrenal gland is also an indirect source of testosterone, both before and after menopause. Giving testosterone to a woman who does not need it can cause problems such as excessive hair growth, acne, and a deepening of the voice. However, women whose menopausal symptoms have failed to respond to estrogen therapy, particularly women whose ovaries have been removed, should consider a trial of Estratest. Your doctor may wish to measure your serum testosterone level to determine whether Estratest is appropriate for you.

CONCLUSION

Estrogen replacement therapy is of value in the treatment of menopausal symptoms and for prevention of osteoporosis. However, because there are risks associated with estrogen, the decision of whether or not to use it should be made on an individual basis, after a detailed discussion with your doctor. Using estriol as a component of your estrogen program may reduce the risk of cancer associated with treatment. In some cases, phytoestrogens derived from foods such as soy may relieve menopausal symptoms. However, it is not known whether phytoestrogens will prevent osteoporosis. In women with testosterone deficiency, addition of testosterone to an estrogen regimen may provide added protection against osteoporosis.

NOTES

1. Gambrell, R. D., Jr. 1992. Complications of estrogen replacement therapy. In *Hormone replacement therapy*, edited by D. P. Swartz, Chapter 9. Baltimore: Williams and Wilkins.

2. Stumpf, P. 1992. Estrogen replacement therapy: current regimens. In *Hormone replacement therapy*, edited by D. P. Swartz, 183. Baltimore: Williams and Wilkins.

3. Follingstad, A. H. 1978. Estriol, the forgotten estrogen? *JAMA* 239:29-30.

4. Tzingounis, V. A., M. F. Aksu, and R. B. Greenblatt. 1978. Estriol in the management of the menopause. *JAMA* 239:1638-1641.

5. Klopper, A. 1980. The risk of endometrial carcinoma from oestrogen therapy of the menopause. *Acta Endocrinol Supp* 233:29-35.

6. Wren, B. G. 1982. Oestriol in the control of postmenopausal symptoms. Preliminary report of a clinical trial. *Med J Aust* 1:176-177.

7. Lemon, H. M., et al. 1966. Reduced estriol excretion in patients with breast cancer prior to endocrine therapy. *JAMA* 196:1128-1136.

8. Lemon, H. M. 1980. Pathophysiologic considerations in the treatment of menopausal patients with oestrogens; the role of oestriol in the prevention of mammary carcinoma. *Acta Endocrinol Suppl* 233:17-27.

9. Lemon, et al., 1128-1136.

10. Ip, C. 1982. Dietary vitamin E intake and mammary carcinogenesis in rats. *Carcinogenesis* 3:1453-1456.

11. London, R. S., et al. 1981. Endocrine parameters and alpha-tocopherol therapy of patients with mammary dysplasia. *Cancer Res* 41:3811–3813.

12. Follingstad, 29–30.

13. Tzingounis, Aksu, and Greenblatt, 1638–1641.

14. Follingstad, 29–30.

15. Wright, J. V., M.D. Personal communication.

16. Tzingounis, Aksu, and Greenblatt. 1638–1641.

17. Adlercreutz, H., et al. 1992. Dietary phyto-oestrogens and the menopause in Japan. *Lancet* 339:1233.

18. Clemetson, C. A. B., et al. 1978. Estrogens in food: The almond mystery. *Int J Gynaecol Obstet* 15:515–521.

19. Elakovich, S. D., and J. M. Hampton. 1984. Analysis of coumestrol, a phytoestrogen, in alfalfa tablets sold for human consumption. *J Agric Food Chem* 32:173–175.

20. Anonymous. 1992. Hormone therapy: Try estrogen/androgen in selected women. *Modern Med* 60(Aug.)21.

15

Progesterone: A Missing Link

MORE IMPORTANT THAN ESTROGEN?

This chapter discusses what could turn out to be the most important breakthrough in decades in relation to osteoporosis treatment and prevention. *Progesterone,* a hormone manufactured by the ovaries, is not only much safer than estrogen, but may also be more effective against osteoporosis. Twenty years from now, scientists may look back and wonder why we focused so much on estrogen, while virtually ignoring progesterone.

When we think of the ovaries losing some of their steam after menopause, we think primarily of a loss of estrogen production. And, when we talk about taking hormones to prevent postmenopausal osteoporosis, we are usually referring to estrogen replacement therapy. As Chapter 14 demonstrates, estrogen therapy does indeed slow the rate of bone loss and reduces the risk of osteoporotic fractures by about 50%. However, estrogen replacement therapy alone is obviously not the entire answer. As many as 1.2 million osteoporotic fractures still occur every year among American women, many of whom are taking estrogen. In addition, because of

141

its risks and side effects a large proportion of women either cannot or will not use estrogen.

OVARIES PRODUCE MORE THAN JUST ESTROGEN

It seems that our focus on estrogen as *the* female hormone has been too limited. We have for some reason ignored the fact that the ovaries of premenopausal women manufacture hormones other than estrogen, and we have failed to consider the possibility that one or more of these other hormones contributes to the association between ovarian function and bone health. There was never any good reason to assume that estrogen is the only ovarian hormone that plays a role in osteoporosis. Perhaps doctors focused on estrogen deficiency because it was so clearly related to menopausal symptoms, such as hot flashes, depression, and vaginal dryness. However, while estrogen replacement therapy is nearly always effective against these troubling menopausal symptoms, estrogen alone is only partially successful as a preventative against osteoporotic fractures. It is logical to assume that if estrogen replacement therapy prevents only 50% of the fractures attributed to postmenopausal osteoporosis, then we are probably missing something very important. There is now reason to believe that one of the factors we have been overlooking is progesterone.

It is well accepted that ovarian hormones play a crucial role in maintaining strong bones. At menopause, when the ovaries become weaker, there is a rapid loss of bone mass for a period of three to eight years, after which bone loss continues at a slower rate. This period of accelerated thinning of the bones occurs at the same time the output of estrogen from the ovaries drops off. However, the production and release of progesterone also declines around the same time. For some reason, doctors have focused on estrogen as the hormone that needs to be "replaced," while assuming that progesterone replacement therapy is not worth considering.

A Reason for Every Hormone

Although that point of view may make sense to drug-oriented doctors who are trained to think in terms of "magic bullets," it is more logical to assume that every hormone manufactured by the ovary is made for a reason. If we choose to support the postmenopausal ovary by administering only one of the hormones involved, we may be doing a poor job of mimicking nature's design.

An example of how most doctors "partition" hormone therapy is the way they treat hypothyroidism (underactive thyroid gland). The generally accepted medication for hypothyroidism is L-thyroxine (Synthroid), which is one of the compounds secreted by our own thyroid gland. Conventional medicine teaches that L-thyroxine and its breakdown product, triiodothyronine (T3), are the only active substances released by the thyroid gland. Doctors, therefore, use L-thyroxine as the sole treatment for hypothyroidism. The problem with that treatment, however, is that the thyroid gland also produces another compound, diiodotyrosine (DIT). Endocrinologists have never figured out what DIT does in the human body, so they proclaim (perhaps ignorantly) that it has no biological activity. It seems rather curious that 38% of all of the organically bound iodine in the thyroid gland is present in the form of DIT. Why would the thyroid gland produce so much of a compound that has no function?

Nutritionally oriented doctors often prefer a natural extract from an animal's thyroid gland over L-thyroxine. This natural form of thyroid hormone, called dessicated thyroid (Armour thyroid), contains L-thyroxine, triiodothyronine, and DIT. It may even contain other, as yet undiscovered, substances that will eventually be found to have an important function. I frequently see patients who are being treated for hypothyroidism with L-thyroxine, but who continue to experience typical hypothyroid symptoms, such as fatigue, depression, cold extremities, fluid retention, and dry skin. However, after switching to an equivalent (or sometimes even less than equivalent) dose of Armour thyroid, their symptoms disappear rapidly.

PROGESTERONE BUILDS BONES

This example supports the concept that every compound secreted by an endocrine gland has a function, even if we have not yet discovered what that function is. We must therefore consider the possibility that the decline in progesterone production that occurs at menopause can have important consequences. That possibility has now been borne out by exciting new research. A growing body of evidence indicates that progesterone is a powerful bone-building hormone and that progesterone replacement therapy could be the next major advance in the battle against osteoporosis. ~~Preliminary results suggest that progesterone is at least as important as, and possibly even more important than, estrogen in preventing and treating postmenopausal osteoporosis.~~

Progesterone is best known as a hormone involved in female reproductive functions. During a woman's fertile years, progesterone helps prepare the uterus to accept a fertilized egg, and then helps maintain the uterus during pregnancy. Its importance in human pregnancy is demonstrated by the fact that women who have previously suffered multiple miscarriages can often deliver a healthy, full-term baby if they are treated with progesterone during their pregnancy. Some doctors also use progesterone with great success to treat premenstrual syndrome. Thus, progesterone is a key hormone in the female endocrine system. It should therefore not be surprising that a condition such as osteoporosis, which involves both women and hormones, could be favorably affected by progesterone.

Life Cycle of Bone Tissue

To understand the possible relationship between progesterone and osteoporosis, it is important to review the life cycle of bone tissue. As discussed in Chapter 3, bone tissue undergoes constant remodeling as old bone is resorbed (dissolved) by special cells called osteoclasts and replaced by new bone, through the action of bone-forming cells called osteoblasts. In healthy premenopausal women the rate of bone resorption and bone formation are closely linked. Thus, if bone resorption accelerates for some reason, then healthy bone will compensate by increasing the amount of new bone formed. As a result of these control mechanisms, the total amount of bone remains relatively constant. This process of remodeling promotes healthier bones, since areas that have been damaged by age or by repetitive stress can be effectively repaired.

After menopause, however, bone resorption and bone formation become uncoupled; that is, they are no longer linked as closely as they were before. While the rate of bone resorption increases significantly after menopause, bone formation fails to keep pace with this rise. In fact, bone formation even declines in some women. Consequently, the healthy process of bone remodeling that takes place prior to menopause is replaced by what might be considered an abnormal state of bone loss.

Estrogen replacement therapy prevents excess bone resorption, slowing the rate of bone loss. However, estrogen therapy does not increase bone formation and, in some cases, actually causes a slight decline. The net effect of estrogen therapy alone, therefore, is less bone remodeling, resulting in a relatively inactive bone mass. The failure of estrogen to reverse the decline in bone formation may be one reason that estrogen prevents only 50% of fractures. As stated, bone that is not actively remodeling and repairing itself can become weakened by the continual effects of physical stress. Fatigue-fractures (hairline cracks resulting from wear and tear) are not adequately repaired and aging bone is not effectively replaced. Inactive bone therefore becomes more susceptible with time to fractures, even if the actual mineral content has not changed substantially. Differences in bone quality probably explain why some women with a given bone mineral content experience numerous fractures, while others with the same bone mineral content have no problems.

Postmenopausal Bone Formation

If there were a way to increase the rate of bone formation after menopause, then postmenopausal women would not only have greater bone mineral content, but stronger and more fracture-resistant bones, as well. Progesterone therapy may be the way to achieve that goal. Jerilynn C. Prior, M.D., of the Division of Endocrinology and Metabolism, University of British Columbia in

Vancouver, has written a comprehensive review of the evidence that progesterone stimulates bone formation.[1] Most interesting is that progesterone binds to osteoblasts, the cells that build new bone. In addition, progesterone interferes with the negative effect that cortisonelike drugs have on osteoblasts. These findings suggest that progesterone acts directly on osteoblasts and may, therefore, promote bone formation.

PROGESTERONE AND BONE LOSS IN FEMALE RUNNERS

Further evidence for a possible role of progesterone in osteoporosis came from a study by Dr. Prior of sixty-six premenopausal women, 21 to 42 years of age.[2] Twenty-one of the women were training for a marathon, twenty-two ran regularly but less intensely, and twenty-three had normal levels of activity. These women were studied because some long-distance runners have accelerated bone loss, in association with amenorrhea (loss of menstruation). All sixty-six women had had two consecutive normal menstrual periods prior to entering the study. During twelve months of observation, the average spinal bone density decreased by about 2% in the group as a whole. However, there were substantial differences in bone loss, depending on whether or not the menstrual cycles remained normal during the study. Among the thirteen women who continued to ovulate and menstruate normally, bone mass actually increased. However, women who developed ovulation disturbances during the study lost 4.2% of their bone mass in one year. While there was no correlation between the rate of bone loss and serum levels of estrogen, there was a close relationship between indicators of progesterone status and bone loss. Women with lower serum levels of progesterone during the luteal phase (the portion of the menstrual cycle in which the most progesterone is released) had higher rates of bone loss than others. Women with shorter luteal phases also had more rapid rates of bone loss.

These results indicate that the loss of bone mass that sometimes occurs in female long-distance runners is related to ovulation disturbances. While estrogen deficiency is sometimes seen in female runners, it does not appear to be an important cause of bone loss in this group. Bone loss was, however, closely correlated with low levels of progesterone. On the other hand, women who had normal ovulatory cycles, and presumably adequate levels of progesterone, actually gained bone mass. It should be noted that long-distance running per se did not cause bone loss. It was only when running was associated with impaired ovulation that a problem developed.

PROGESTOGEN THERAPY AND OSTEOPOROSIS

So far, we have learned that progesterone plays a role in bone formation, that progesterone deficiency is associated with bone loss in long-distance runners, and that progesterone levels decline after menopause. Although this evidence is circumstantial it suggests that progesterone therapy may be beneficial in osteoporosis.

Progesteronelike compounds, known as *progestogens,* have been used with some success to treat osteoporosis. In one study, ten elderly men with asthma who had developed osteoporosis from long-term prednisone therapy were given a progestogen (medroxyprogesterone acetate) plus calcium supplements. Five men with similar problems (control group) received no calcium or hormones. After one year, bone density in the treated group had increased by 17%, compared to a 15% decline in the control group. This degree of improvement is substantial, far greater than the results obtained by conventional treatments for osteoporosis. Although the men also received calcium, the dramatic improvements were almost certainly due to the progestogen since calcium therapy is of only minimal benefit for individuals who develop bone loss from cortisone-like drugs.

Progestogens have also shown promise in the prevention and treatment of postmenopausal osteoporosis. In one study, fourteen osteoporotic women to whom estrogen therapy could not be given because of cancer or other reasons were treated with a progestogen for nine months. During that time, there was a 4% increase in bone mass compared to an expected decline of 2 to 4% per year.[3] In another study, thirty-six postmenopausal women were given either a progestogen (medroxyprogesterone acetate) alone, estrogen alone, or both hormones. Each woman also received a calcium supplement. The progestogen was about as effective as estrogen in preventing bone loss. Women who received both hormones had slightly greater bone mass than those who received either hormone alone.[4] Other studies have produced similar results.

Progestogens (such as Provera) are now routinely used along with estrogen replacement therapy. The main reason for adding a progestogen is that it eliminates the excess risk of uterine cancer that results from using estrogen alone. An apparent added benefit of adding a progestogen to estrogen replacement therapy is that bone mass is more effectively preserved.

NATURAL PROGESTERONE SUPERIOR TO PROGESTOGENS

This story might have ended here since many doctors are already using progestogens. However, the story cannot end here because the medical profession is still overlooking an important point— namely, that progesterone and progestogens are not the same thing. While progestogens are similar to progesterone in both structure and function, there are also fundamental differences both in their biological activity and in their toxicity. Since even small changes in the structure of steroid hormones can greatly alter their effects, it is possible that progestogens are less effective bone builders than progesterone. Exciting new research discussed next indicates that progesterone is, indeed, considerably more potent in this respect than its synthetic counterparts. Furthermore, while progestogens can cause any one of a long list of adverse reactions natural progesterone is almost entirely free of side effects. For these reasons, the story will be complete only after the medical profession has taken a serious look at natural progesterone for postmenopausal women.

Progesterone Poorly Absorbed

Progestogens were originally synthesized as alternatives to progesterone, which is thought to be relatively ineffective when given by mouth. Part of the problem with orally administered progesterone is that it is not efficiently absorbed across the intestinal tract. The other problem is that substances absorbed orally must pass through the liver before they enter the body's general circulation. In the case of progesterone, much of what is absorbed is metabolized by the liver into inactive breakdown products before it has a chance to act elsewhere in the body. Consequently, progesterone is usually administered by intramuscular injection or by rectal or vaginal suppository, a fact that limits its acceptability.

Progestogens versus Progesterone

Scientists therefore searched for compounds structurally similar to progesterone that could be absorbed when taken by mouth. A number of such compounds have been synthesized; they mimic the action of progesterone in their ability to promote withdrawal bleeding in the uterus. These progestogens are effective and convenient for use in birth control pills, for helping to synchronize abnormal menstrual cycles, and to counteract the cancer-promoting effect of estrogen replacement therapy in postmenopausal women. However, because of their structural differences the actions of progesterone and progestogens differ significantly in other respects.

Indeed, progestogens exhibit some actions that would be considered antagonistic to those of progesterone.[5] Whereas progesterone causes a reduction in salt and water retention, progestogens do the opposite. That is why some women who are taking birth control pills or a postmenopausal hormone combination containing a progestogen experience bloating and fluid retention. Whereas progesterone aids in conception and helps maintain pregnancy, progestogens inhibit ovulation and are therefore used for birth control. Administering progestogens has been shown to lower the blood

level of progesterone. Some women apparently have a subtle progesterone deficiency that becomes more severe when they take a
progestogen. This fact may explain why many women who have had
severe side effects from birth control pills or from other hormone
regimens containing progestogens improve when they receive natural progesterone. In fact, one of the clues in a medical history that
predicts a beneficial response to progesterone is a history of intolerance to progestogens.

In addition to its antiprogesterone effects, progestogens may
cause a number of other side effects including mental depression,
weight gain, nausea, insomnia, abnormal vaginal bleeding, breast
tenderness, and various types of skin rashes. Progestogens also occasionally cause more serious or even life-threatening complications, such as cholestatic jaundice (a form of liver disease),
thrombophlebitis (blood clots in the veins) or pulmonary embo-
lism (blood clots in the lungs). Natural progesterone, on the other
hand, is almost entirely free of adverse side effects.

PROGESTERONE TREATMENT OF OSTEOPOROSIS

It is clear from this evidence that progesterone is safer than progestogens and that, at least in theory, might be more effective against
osteoporosis. However, routine use of progesterone had been limited by the lack of a convenient form in which to administer it. That
limitation was overcome in the 1970s when it was discovered that
progesterone can be absorbed through the skin into the
bloodstream.

The Lee Study

In 1981, John R. Lee, M.D., from Sebastopol, California, became
interested in the potential value of natural progesterone. He began
what is now a landmark study of progesterone in the treatment of
osteoporosis.[7] One hundred postmenopausal women, ages 38 to 83
(average, 65.2), applied a cream containing 3% progesterone to
their skin instead of taking the usual medroxyprogesterone acetate

(Provera) by mouth. Most of the women had already become shorter as a result of one or more spontaneous vertebral fractures. Conjugated estrogens such as Premarin (0.3 to 0.625 mg/day; three weeks
per month) were given when appropriate. However, more than one-
third of the women did not receive estrogen because they had
medical conditions that rendered estrogen therapy too dangerous,
such as obesity, varicose veins, elevated cholesterol or triglycerides,
fibrocystic breast disease, history of breast cancer, endometrial
cancer, clotting disorders, or thromboembolism.

Each participant in the study applied the progesterone cream
at night for twelve consecutive days per month or during the last
two weeks of estrogen use. This regimen was followed for a minimum of three years. To promote efficient absorption of progesterone the cream was applied to softer areas of the skin, such as under
the arms or on the neck or face, and these application sites were
rotated. The usual dose was one-third to one-half ounce of cream
per month. In addition to using progesterone, the women were
advised to include leafy green vegetables in their diet, to minimize
the consumption of cigarettes, alcohol, and red meat, and to exercise three times a week. They were also urged to take various nutritional supplements, including calcium, vitamin D, and vitamin C.

The Results

In this group of one hundred patients treated with progesterone for
at least three years, aches and pains in the muscles and bones
disappeared, height loss was stabilized, and no further osteoporotic
fractures occurred. These results by themselves were encouraging,
but the most dramatic effect of progesterone therapy was on bone
mineral density. In 63 of the 100 women in the study, bone density
of the the lumbar spine was measured by dual photon absorptiometry every three to six months (the other thirty-seven women could
not afford the cost of the test, which is usually not covered by
medical insurance). The natural history of osteoporosis would have
predicted an average bone loss of 4.5% among Lee's patients. However, of the sixty-three women in whom bone density was assessed,

not a single one lost bone mass. In fact, the opposite was true. Every one of the sixty-three women treated with progesterone had an increase in bone mass. Furthermore, in many cases this increase was substantial, far greater than what has been achieved with other osteoporosis therapies.

Dr. Lee frequently observed a 10% increase in bone mineral density after the first 6 to 12 months of therapy. Some patients even had a 20 to 25% increase during the first year. After the first twelve months of treatment, bone density continued to increase by about 3 to 5% per year until it stabilized at the levels seen in healthy thirty-five-year-old women. In the group as a whole, average bone density increased by 15.4%. The beneficial effects of progesterone were not affected by age; seventy-year-old women often had the same increase in bone density as did younger women. The probability of improvement was most closely related to initial lumbar bone density. Women with the lowest initial bone densities had the greatest increases, whereas those with initially dense bones did not show as much improvement. It is encouraging that the best results occurred in women who needed them the most, and that progesterone can apparently help any woman, no matter how far her bones have deteriorated.

Side Effects Almost Nonexistent

Many of the women receiving progesterone therapy commented that their mobility and energy level improved and that their low sex drive returned to normal. Side effects were almost nonexistent. One woman had slight vaginal spotting after one cycle of treatment and was found to have uterine cancer. No other side effects were seen.

Effects on Fractures

As mentioned, not one of the one hundred women in the study suffered a new osteoporotic fracture. Since most of the women had already had one or more spontaneous vertebral crush fractures and many were becoming progressively shorter, it is remarkable that no further fractures or height loss occurred. Additional evidence of the effectiveness of progesterone was seen in three women who did suffer fractures, not because of osteoporosis, but as a result of trauma. One eighty-year-old woman fractured her knee in an automobile accident; another (in her seventies) fell while hiking and broke her arm; a third woman broke her arm after falling down the stairs. All three of these fractures healed well and the treating orthopedists commented on the excellent bone structure of these women.

Impact of Estrogen

Another noteworthy finding in Lee's study was that estrogen did not enhance the bone-building effect of progesterone. In other words, women who received both estrogen and progesterone had no better results than women who received progesterone alone. If Lee's observations are correct, then osteoporosis can be effectively reversed by progesterone alone, regardless of whether or not estrogen is used. As mentioned earlier in this chapter, the main effect of estrogen is to inhibit bone resorption, while the primary action of progesterone is to promote bone formation. It is possible that bone formation is a more important part of the equation than bone resorption, where postmenopausal osteoporosis is concerned. The fact that progesterone can be converted to some extent into estrogen within the body may also explain the observation that progesterone alone is effective. Having found that estrogen does not improve the results of progesterone therapy, Lee no longer prescribes estrogen for prevention of osteoporosis, although he still uses it to treat hot flashes and vaginal dryness.

More Study Needed

So far, no other researchers have followed up on Lee's report. I have informally surveyed some my colleagues in nutritional medicine and have found that many of them are prescribing natural progesterone. However, none of these doctors have monitored their results with repeated bone density studies. Hopefully, we will have more information about this important treatment within the next few years.

SAFETY OF PROGESTERONE

The results reported by Lee are substantially better than those obtained with any other treatment for osteoporosis. The absence of side effects is also very encouraging. Further, while progestogens frequently cause adverse changes in cholesterol levels progesterone had no such effect. Nor is there evidence that progesterone poses any cancer risk. On the contrary, in a study on guinea pigs administering progesterone prevented the precancerous changes in the cervical lining caused by estrogen therapy. In addition, of seventeen women with cervical cancer who were treated with progesterone eleven showed evidence of tumor regression.[6] Progesterone has also been used with some success to treat vaginal cancer in women exposed to DES (stilbestrol).

One important question about progesterone is whether it can prevent estrogen-induced uterine cancer, as progestogens do. Christiane Northrup, M.D., an expert on women's health, has investigated that question in the course of treating more then 200 postmenopausal women with progesterone cream. According to Northrup, breakthrough bleeding is uncommon in women receiving low-dose estrogen plus natural progesterone. In cases where breakthrough bleeding did occur, endometrial biopsies showed no evidence of endometrial hyperplasia, a precancerous change in the uterus.[8] However, some doctors are concerned that progesterone cream may not always be strong enough to counterbalance the carcinogenic effect of estrogen. If you have a uterus and are taking estrogen, consult your physician about the appropriate hormone combination to use.

CONCLUSION

Natural progesterone appears to be extremely effective for preventing and treating osteoporosis. In contrast to synthetic progestogens which have many side effects and risks, progesterone is quite safe. The use of progesterone may eliminate the need for estrogen replacement therapy in many cases. If Lee's results are confirmed by additional studies, then we will have achieved an important breakthrough in the battle against osteoporosis. Although Lee's work is now several years old, no one has yet attempted to duplicate his findings. Because of the important implications of his work, follow-up studies should be a top research priority.

NOTES

1. Prior, J. C. 1990. Progesterone as a bone-trophic hormone. *Endocrine Rev* 11:386–398.

2. Prior, J. C., et al. 1990. Spinal bone loss and ovulatory disturbances. *N Engl J Med* 323:1221–1227.

3. McCann, J., and N. Horwitz. 1987. Provera alone builds bone. *Med Tribune,* 22 July, 4–5.

4. McNeeley, S. G., Jr., et al. 1991. Prevention of osteoporosis by medroxyprogesterone acetate in postmenopausal women. *Int J Gynecol Obstet* 34:253–256.

5. Dalton, K. 1984. *The premenstrual syndrome and progesterone therapy.* Chicago: Year Book Medical Publishers, Inc.

6. Hertz, R., et al. 1951. Observations on the effect of progesterone on carcinoma of the cervix. *J Natl Cancer Inst* 11:867–873.

7. Lee, J. R. 1991. Osteoporosis reversal: the role of progesterone. *Int Clin Nutr Rev* 10(3):384–391. Lee, J. R. 1990. Osteoporosis reversal with transdermal progesterone. *Lancet* 336:1327. Lee, J. R. 1991. Is natural progesterone the missing link in osteoporosis prevention and treatment? *Med Hypotheses* 35:316–318.

8. Northrup, C. Personal communication.

16

DHEA: The Hormone That "Does It All"

Many people have a negative attitude about hormones. For them, the thought of taking hormones conjures up images of growing pimples and excessive hair, getting fat or depressed, or, worst of all, developing cancer. Hormones are small molecules which have a powerful influence on every cell in your body. However, we seem to be most aware of them when they are out of balance.

Hormones are actually not bad molecules at all. In fact, without them you would not be healthy, or even alive. Problems occur when hormones get out of balance—either too much or too little of one, or an improper ratio of one to another. On the other hand, hormones have been used therapeutically for many different conditions and are some of the most powerful biologic agents known.

A hormone produced by the adrenal glands has until recently received little attention. However, new evidence suggests that this hormone is so beneficial for so many different conditions that it may turn out to be the most important medical advance of the decade. I am not talking about cortisone, that double-edged sword which has saved the lives of many people, but which can also cause severe side effects including osteoporosis. I am talking about dehy-droepiandrosterone (DHEA), another adrenal hormone, which may turn out to be as much of a "wonder drug" as cortisone has been, with the added advantage of being relatively free of side effects. One should always be skeptical about a new treatment that is claimed to be good for "almost everything." However, we cannot ignore the rapidly expanding body of scientific research which suggests that DHEA may be helpful for preventing and treating a wide range of medical conditions.

DHEA CHEMISTRY

DHEA is a steroid hormone which is structurally similar to other steroid hormones (such as estrogen, progesterone, and testoster-one), but which possesses its own spectrum of biologic effects. Scientists have known for years that DHEA is secreted by the adrenal gland and that there is a greater quantity of this hormone produced than of any other adrenal steroid. However, until recently, no one knew why the adrenals make DHEA or what its function is in the body. As it was known that DHEA can be converted into other hormones, including estrogen and testosterone, scientists assumed that DHEA is merely a "buffer hormone," a reservoir upon which the adrenals could draw to produce more of these other hormones. However, scientists have recently shown that cells contain specific DHEA receptors, the sole function of which is to bind DHEA. That finding strongly suggests that DHEA is more than just a buffer hor-mone, that it has functions of its own in the body.

THERAPEUTIC VALUE OF DHEA

Current research suggests that DHEA may be of value in preventing and treating cardiovascular disease, high cholesterol, diabetes, obe-sity, cancer, Alzheimer's disease, other memory disturbances, im-mune system disorders including acquired immunodeficiency syndrome (AIDS), and chronic fatigue. DHEA may also enhance the body's immune response to viral and bacterial infections. Perhaps most interesting, DHEA is currently being investigated as an anti-aging hormone. And, of particular interest to readers of this book, DHEA may also be of value in preventing and treating osteoporosis.

When one reads the list of conditions for which DHEA is currently being investigated, it tends to read somewhat like a snake oil salesperson's compendium. Nevertheless, it is not unreasonable to suggest that a substance that occurs naturally in the body could have such a wide range of seemingly unrelated effects. Deficiency of vitamin C, for example, can cause fatigue, depression, impaired immune system function, arthritis, heart and blood vessel disease, poor wound healing, bone abnormalities, bleeding gums, and other problems. Magnesium deficiency can also cause a myriad of disorders, as discussed in Chapter 5. Why, then, should it not be possible that a deficiency of a hormone could result in a broad spectrum of dysfunctions? A brief summary of some of the research published on DHEA is presented next, to give you a perspective on how powerful this substance appears to be.

Diabetes

A certain inbred strain of mice has a genetic disorder that causes them to develop diabetes. Their pancreatic beta cells, those cells in the pancreas that make insulin, are also spontaneously destroyed during the course of their lifetime. When this strain of mice was given 0.4% DHEA in their diet, the diabetes was rapidly reversed and the beta cells were preserved. In a study of other animals without this genetic disorder, DHEA reduced the severity of diabetes resulting from administering the diabetes-inducing chemical, streptozotocin.[1]

Heart Disease

A study published several years ago in the *New England Journal of Medicine* showed that DHEA may play a role in preventing heart disease.[2] Plasma levels of DHEA-S (the "S" stands for sulfate) were measured in 242 men, ages 50 to 79. DHEA-S, a byproduct of DHEA, is easier to measure and provides a rough estimate of DHEA levels.

In men with a history of heart disease, DHEA-S levels were significantly lower than in those with no history of heart disease. Furthermore, among men with healthy hearts, those who had low levels of DHEA were 3.3 times more likely to die of heart disease during the next twelve years than were those with normal DHEA levels. Administering DHEA has also been shown to lower serum LDL-cholesterol, the "bad" form of cholesterol, which is associated with heart disease.[3] These results raise the possibility that in individuals with low DHEA levels supplementing with DHEA may help prevent heart disease.

Obesity

Animal studies suggest that DHEA may be effective in treating obesity. In a strain of mice that has a genetic predisposition to obesity, administering DHEA at a dose of 500 mg/kg of body weight, three times a week, prevented the development of obesity. DHEA did not cause any toxic effects and did not suppress appetite, indicating that its effect was to speed up the metabolism.[4] In another study, administering DHEA (0.6% of the diet) decreased body weight and body fat in both lean and obese Zucker rats. The decrease in body fat was primarily due to a decrease in the number of fat cells in lean rats and to decreases in both the number and size of fat cells in obese rats.[5]

Cancer

In contrast to estrogen, which may promote cancer under certain circumstances, DHEA shows promise as an anticancer agent. In a strain of mice that develops spontaneous breast cancer, long-term administration of DHEA prevented the cancer from occurring.[6] Treatment of mice with DHEA also delayed the appearance of colon tumors resulting from administering the carcinogen 1,2-dimethylhydrazine.[7] Administering DHEA also inhibited the development of liver cancer in rats treated with chemical carcinogens.[8]

Other studies indicate that there is an association between

DHEA levels and human breast cancer. In one study, urinary excretion of DHEA was below normal in a group of premenopausal women with breast cancer.[9] Other researchers confirmed that DHEA levels are low in premenopausal breast cancer patients, but found that some postmenopausal women with breast cancer had elevated DHEA levels.[10] It appeared that the low levels in the premenopausal patients were due primarily to decreased production, while the elevated levels in the postmenopausal patients were due to delayed breakdown. Whatever the reason for the changes, these studies suggest a possible role for DHEA in the prevention or treatment of at least some cases of breast cancer.

Autoimmune Diseases

Conditions in which the immune system mistakenly attacks the body's own tissues are called *autoimmune diseases.* Various types of arthritis, systemic lupus erythematosus (SLE), inflammatory bowel disease (ulcerative colitis and Crohn's disease), and other inflammatory or connective tissue disorders are considered autoimmune diseases. Many other common conditions including diabetes, hypertension, and heart disease, are thought to have an autoimmune component.

Studies in animals suggest that DHEA may have a beneficial effect on the process of autoimmune attack. The New Zealand Black mouse is a strain of mice that spontaneously develops an autoimmune syndrome resembling SLE. Administering DHEA to these animals prevented the kidney failure and the hemolytic anemia associated with this syndrome.[11]

DHEA has been shown to increase the production of interleukin-2, a component of the immune system which is consistently decreased in individuals with SLE. Because of these intriguing observations, Dr. Jim McGuire, Associate Professor of Medicine at Stanford University of Medicine, is currently conducting a clinical trial of DHEA in patients with SLE. DHEA is also being tested in patients with multiple sclerosis. Preliminary findings indicate that DHEA produces a significant improvement in stamina and in sense of well being in people suffering from multiple sclerosis.[12]

Dr. Davis Lamson, a private practitioner in Kent, Washington, has also been seeing some exciting results with DHEA in various autoimmune disorders. He finds that serum levels of DHEA are often toward the lower end of normal or below normal in people with rheumatoid arthritis or ulcerative colitis. Lamson has given DHEA to six patients with ulcerative colitis who had failed to respond to a combination of conventional therapy and nutritional treatments. In all six cases, the bleeding, diarrhea, and overall condition improved. Dr. Lamson has also found DHEA therapy to be of value in treating rheumatoid arthritis and other forms of arthritis, as long as the initial DHEA level is on the low side.[13]

AIDS

Another immune system–related condition in which DHEA may play a role is acquired immunodeficiency syndrome (AIDS). DHEA has been reported to inhibit the replication of HIV, the virus believed to cause AIDS.[14] In addition, this hormone has been shown to enhance the immune response to viral infections. Furthermore, DHEA levels are reduced in people infected with HIV, with these levels declining even more as the disease progresses to full-blown AIDS.[15] In a recent study, 108 HIV-positive men with marginally low helper T-cell counts (between 200 and 499) were observed. Men with serum DHEA levels below normal were 2.34 times as likely to progress to AIDS as were those with normal DHEA levels.[16] These studies provide evidence that a deficiency of DHEA occurs in individuals with HIV infection and that this deficiency may be one of the factors contributing to immune system failure.

Chronic Fatigue Syndrome (CFS)

This debilitating condition was first described in the early 1980s and is becoming increasingly prevalent among young adults and middle-aged Americans. The cause of this problem has not been identified, although several viruses are suspected. Conventional treatment has so far been unsatisfactory. Nutrition-oriented doctors have had some success treating CFS with allergy diets, thyroid hormones, nutrient injections (particularly magnesium and B-vitamins) and other treatments. During the past several years, a growing number of doctors have begun giving DHEA to individuals whose levels are low-normal or below normal. In some cases, this treatment produces definite improvement in energy level, stamina, and general well being.

Aging

Preliminary results in mice suggest that DHEA may retard the aging process. Animals treated with this hormone looked younger, had glossier coats, and less gray hair than control animals.[17] In humans, serum levels of DHEA are known to decline with age; the levels in seventy-year-old individuals are only about 20% as high as those in young adults. This age-related decline is not known to occur with any of the other adrenal steroids. It has therefore been suggested that some of the manifestations of aging may be caused by DHEA deficiency. In my experience, some elderly people who suffer from weakness, muscle wasting, tremulousness, and other signs of aging experience noticeable improvements within several weeks of beginning small doses of DHEA (such as 5 to 15 mg/day).

DHEA: AN OVARIAN HORMONE

Osteoporosis is another one of the manifestations of aging, and there is evidence that the decline in DHEA levels may be a factor in age-related bone loss. DHEA is manufactured by the adrenal glands, but it is also one of the four major hormones produced by the ovaries; the others are estrogen, progesterone, and testosterone. In previous chapters, we have shown that both estrogen and progesterone have beneficial effects on osteoporosis—the former by inhibiting bone resorption, and the latter by stimulating bone formation. Testosterone has also been shown to improve osteoporosis.[18]

It would be surprising, therefore, if the fourth major ovarian hormone, DHEA, did not also play a role in the ovary–osteoporosis connection.

In fact, when one looks at the various biochemical effects of DHEA, they tend to read like the "who's who of osteoporosis prevention." First, one of the breakdown products of DHEA, a compound called 5-androstene-3β, 17β-diol, is known to bind strongly to estrogen receptors.[19] Therefore DHEA, like estrogen, might inhibit bone resorption. Second, there is evidence that androgens (a class of hormones that includes DHEA and testosterone) stimulate bone formation and calcium absorption.[20] DHEA might, therefore, augment the bone-building effect of progesterone. As far as we can tell, DHEA is the only hormone that appears capable of both inhibiting bone resorption and stimulating bone formation.

DHEA Increases Levels of Other Hormones

A third function of DHEA, that of a precursor hormone, almost certainly results in a beneficial influence on osteoporosis. DHEA can be converted by the body into other hormones including estrogen and testosterone, both of which play a role in prevention of bone loss. In a study of postmenopausal women, administering DHEA increased serum levels of both testosterone and estrogens (estradiol and estrone).[21]

Finally, DHEA may be capable of raising the levels of progesterone. Although DHEA is not converted directly into progesterone, it may, through a feedback mechanism, indirectly increase the production of progesterone. Both DHEA and progesterone are produced from the same precursor hormone, pregnenolone. If enough DHEA is present, then pregnenolone will be converted primarily to progesterone, rather than to DHEA.

These multiple functions of DHEA seem rather impressive. Not only does this hormone apparently have a direct effect on both resorption and formation of bone, but it can also increase the levels of the other major hormonal "players"—namely, estrogen, progesterone, and testosterone. Furthermore, there is no need to worry that taking DHEA will cause cancer because the evidence suggests that it actually prevents cancer.

DHEA AND OSTEOPOROSIS

In view of the exciting potential of DHEA, it is surprising that no one has until now tested the effect of this hormone on bone mass and fracture incidence. Several such trials were in progress as of January 1993, and the results of these studies should be available within a year or two. The scientific community got a late start with DHEA: It was only a few years ago that DHEA began its transformation from the hormone with no function into the hormone that "does it all." Nevertheless, a number of additional observations support the theoretical benefits of DHEA in osteoporosis.

Effects of Falling DHEA Levels

It has been shown that menopause is associated with a reduction in DHEA levels. In one study, the average plasma level of DHEA (ng/100 ml) was 542 in premenopausal women, 197 in postmenopausal women, and only 126 in women whose ovaries had been surgically removed.[22] In a group of women between the ages of 55 and 85 years, there was a significant correlation between serum levels of DHEA (measured as DHEA-S) and bone density of the vertebral spine.[23] In other words, women with higher levels of DHEA had greater bone mass than those with lower DHEA levels.

Impact of Aging

Since bone mass and serum DHEA both decline with advancing age, one cannot be certain that falling DHEA levels are actually the cause of reduced bone mass. However, there is evidence that aging alone cannot explain the relationship between DHEA levels and bone mass. In a recent study of Belgian women significant correlations were found between bone mineral content and DHEA levels (measured as DHEA-S), even after correcting for the effects of age.[24] In another study, serum DHEA levels were significantly lower in forty-nine women with osteoporosis than in women of similar age without osteoporosis. Although DHEA levels declined with age in both groups of women, those with osteoporosis had lower levels of DHEA at all ages.[25] These studies support the proposed role of DHEA in maintaining bone mass.

DHEA, Rheumatoid Arthritis, and Corticosteroids

DHEA levels have also been found to be low in women with rheumatoid arthritis, a condition frequently associated with osteoporosis. In a study of forty-nine postmenopausal women with rheumatoid arthritis, DHEA levels (measured as DHEA-S) were significantly lower than in healthy controls.[26] DHEA levels were reduced to a greater extent in women taking corticosteroids (cortisonelike drugs) for their arthritis than in those who were not. That finding is not surprising, since administering these drugs is known to reduce the levels of adrenal androgens such as DHEA.[27] However, DHEA levels were also significantly reduced in arthritic women who were not receiving corticosteroids. In this group of forty-nine women, DHEA levels correlated significantly with bone mineral density of the neck of the femur (a bone in the hip) and the spine. The serum level of DHEA was able to predict bone mineral density, even after corticosteroid therapy was taken into account. This study suggests that DHEA might be of benefit to people with rheumatoid arthritis.

Corticosteroids are known to be an important cause of osteoporosis, perhaps, in part, because they deplete DHEA. Would simultaneous administration of DHEA inhibit some of the side effects of corticosteroids, including osteoporosis? Our natural adrenal secretions contain both of these hormones, and nature usually does things for a reason. Animal studies suggest that DHEA does, in fact, modulate some of the effects of corticosteroids.[28]

Supplementing with DHEA might prevent the osteoporosis that so often develops in individuals with rheumatoid arthritis, particularly in those who are taking corticosteroids. In addition, DHEA may impact positively on the arthritic process itself. According to Dr. Lamson, who has given DHEA to several arthritic patients with low serum levels of DHEA, this treatment often relieves pain and morning stiffness, increases strength, and reduces the need for anti-inflammatory medication. In a study of forty-five postmenopausal women being treated with corticosteroids, administering DHEA (20 mg/day) resulted in an increased sense of well-being, with no side effects.[29]

Osteoporosis: Additional Evidence

An additional clue to the relationship between DHEA and bones comes from a study of individuals with Addison's disease, also known as adrenal insufficiency. This condition results from a failure of the adrenal cortex to produce adequate amounts of adrenal hormones. Bone mineral density measurements at the radius (a bone in the forearm) showed normal values in premenopausal women with Addison's disease. However, in postmenopausal women with this disorder there was a dramatic loss of bone which exceeded the typical postmenopausal decline. This accelerated bone loss was associated with a profound reduction in plasma DHEA levels, which averaged 94% lower than those of healthy postmenopausal women. Plasma concentrations of estrogen and testosterone, two of the by-products of DHEA, were also reduced.[30]

These findings strongly suggest that DHEA secreted by the adrenal cortex plays an important role in maintaining bone mass in postmenopausal women. In premenopausal women with Addison's disease, enough DHEA is apparently made by the ovaries to compensate for the weak adrenal glands. That most likely explains why these women do not develop osteoporosis. After menopause, however, when ovarian production of DHEA slows down the adrenal glands are not capable of taking over and a marked deficiency of DHEA results. It is quite possible that giving DHEA to postmenopausal women with adrenal insufficiency would prevent the accelerated bone loss that these women experience.

DHEA and Calcium Metabolism

Until the clinical trials now in progress are completed, we will not know for sure just how much DHEA can do to prevent osteoporosis. Hopefully, these trials will be completed within a year or two. However, experiments performed more than fifteen years ago by Dr. Hollo, a Hungarian researcher, provide a hint of how the newer studies may turn out. Hollo, like other later investigators, found that plasma levels of DHEA-S were significantly lower in postmenopausal women with osteoporosis than in matched controls. He also found another abnormality in these women; when they were given calcium by intravenous injection, the calcium level in their bloodstream remained elevated for an unusually long period of time. However, after receiving DHEA-S (100 mg/day by mouth for seven days) their calcium metabolism returned to normal.[31]

THE FUTURE OF DHEA THERAPY

How Much to Take?

The evidence presented in this chapter provides a strong case for using DHEA as part of an overall osteoporosis prevention and treatment program. More research is needed to answer the many questions that remain. We do not know at the present time the optimal dose of DHEA. Practitioners using DHEA are typically prescribing 3 to 30 mg/day, although much larger doses are being given to patients with cancer, AIDS, and other serious conditions.

We still lack a clear understanding of who should receive DHEA, or when it should be started. It seems logical to consider a small dose of DHEA (say, 3 to 5 mg/day) in the early postmenopausal period, and a larger dose (perhaps 5 to 15 mg/day) in later years, when adrenal output declines. Commercial laboratories can measure blood levels of DHEA and DHEA-S. These measurements may provide a crude estimate of DHEA status, but they cannot predict with certainty who will benefit from treatment or what the dosage should be. Jonathan V. Wright, M.D., a leading authority in nutritional medicine, has observed that absence of hair on the lower third of the legs is suggestive of DHEA deficiency.

Fortunately, DHEA appears to be quite safe. Dosages as high as 1,600 mg/day have been given for periods of twenty-eight days without any serious side effects, although mild abnormalities of blood sugar metabolism occurred in some cases.[32] It is probable that much lower doses, perhaps in the range of 3 to 30 mg/day, are needed for prevention and treatment of osteoporosis. Minor side effects, such as acne or a slight increase in hair growth on the arms and legs, may occasionally occur when DHEA is taken.

Effects on Other Hormones

We also need to know exactly how DHEA therapy affects the requirements for estrogen and progesterone. One of the most important principles of hormone therapy is to try to mimic as closely as possible the natural glandular secretions. In the case of postmenopausal hormone replacement therapy, that would include the use of estrogen, progesterone, and DHEA (although the ovaries also manufacture testosterone, production of this hormone usually does not decline after menopause). It is likely that combined use of all three of these hormones would provide the best results, while at the same time permitting the use of lower doses of each of the individual hormones. Lamson has found, for example, that supplementing with DHEA sometimes enhances the effectiveness of estrogen against menopausal symptoms such as hot flashes. Christiane Northrup, M.D., has found a similar interaction between estrogen and natural progesterone.[33] However, as far as I am aware, no one has yet studied the effects of giving all three of these hormones at the same time.

Nonpatentable Therapeutic Potential

At the present time, most physicians are unaware of the importance of DHEA. Furthermore, DHEA is available at only a handful of pharmacies in the United States. As is typical of most natural, nonpatentable substances, the pharmaceutical industry has had no interest in putting its research funds or promotional dollars into DHEA. Nevertheless, as the research on DHEA continues to come in a growing number of doctors are becoming interested in the therapeutic potential of this "hormone that does it all." Until we know more about this exciting substance, we should use it with caution and should monitor closely for possible long-term side effects.

NOTES

1. Coleman, D. L., E. H. Leiter, and R. W. Schwizer. 1982. Therapeutic effects of dehydroepiandrosterone (DHEA) in diabetic mice. *Diabetes* 31:830–833.

2. Barrett-Connor, E., K-T. Khaw, and S. S. C. Yen. 1986. A prospective study of dehydroepiandrosterone sulfate, mortality, and cardiovascular disease. *N Engl J Med* 315:1519–1524.

3. Regelson, W., R. Loria, and M. Kalimi. 1988. Hormonal intervention: "Buffer hormones" or "state dependency." The role of dehydroepiandrosterone (DHEA), thyroid hormone, estrogen and hypophysectomy in aging. *Ann NY Acad Sci* 521:260–273.

4. Yen, T. T., et al. 1977. Prevention of obesity in Avy/a mice by dehydroepiandrosterone. *Lipids* 12:409–413.

5. Cleary, M. P, A. Shepherd, and B. Jenks. 1984. Effect of dehydroepiandrosterone on growth in lean and obese Zucker rats. *J Nutr* 114:1242–1251.

6. Schwartz, A. G. 1979. Inhibition of spontaneous breast cancer formation in female C3H(Avy/a) mice by long-term treatment with dehydroepiandrosterone. *Cancer Res* 39:1129–1132.

7. Nyce, J. W., et al. 1984. Inhibition of 1,2-dimethylhydrazine-induced colon tumorigenesis in Balb/c mice by dehydroepiandrosterone. *Carcinogenesis* 5:57–62.

8. Mayer, D., E. Weber, and P. Bannasch. 1990. Modulation of liver carcinogenesis by dehydroepiandrosterone. In *The biological role of dehydroepiandrosterone,* edited by M. Kalimi and W. Regelson, 361–385. New York: de Gruyter.

9. Arguelles, A. E., et al. 1973. Endocrine profiles and breast cancer. *Lancet* 1:165–168.

10. Zumoff, B., et al. 1981. Abnormal 24-hr mean plasma concentrations of dehydroisoandrosterone and dehydroisoandrosterone sulfate in women with primary operable breast cancer. *Cancer Res* 41:3360–3363.

11. Regelson, Loria, and Kalimi, 260–273.

12. Calabrese, V. P., E. R. Isaacs, and W. Regelson. 1990. Dehydroepiandrosterone

in multiple sclerosis: positive effects on the fatigue syndrome in a non-randomized study. In *The biological role of dehydroepiandrosterone,* edited by M. Kalimi and W. Regelson, 95–100. New York: de Gruyter.

13. Lamson, D., Dr. Personal communication.

14. Jacobson, M. A., et al. 1991. Decreased serum dehydroepiandrosterone is associated with an increased progression of human immunodeficiency virus infection in men with CD4 cell counts of 200–499. *J Infect Dis* 164:864–868.

15. Merril, C. R., M. G. Harrington, and T. Sunderland. 1990. Reduced plasma dehydroepiandrosterone concentrations in HIV infection and Alzheimer's disease. In *The biological role of dehydroepiandrosterone,* edited by M. Kalimi and W. Regelson, 101–105. New York: de Gruyter.

16. Jacobson, et al., 864–868.

17. Anonymous. 1981. Antiobesity drug may counter aging. *Science News* 19(3):39.

18. Anonymous. 1992. Hormone therapy: Try estrogen/androgen in selected women. *Modern Med* 60(August):21.

19. Taelman, P., et al. 1989. Persistence of increased bone resorption and possible role of dehydroepiandrosterone as a bone metabolism determinant in osteoporotic women in late post-menopause. *Maturitas* 11:65–73.

20. Ibid.

21. Mortola, J. F., and S. S. C. Yen. 1990. The effects of oral dehydroepiandrosterone on endocrine-metabolic parameters in postmenopausal women. *J Clin Endocrinol Metab* 71:696–704.

22. Monroe, S. E., and K. M. J. Menon. 1977. Changes in reproductive hormone secretion during the climacteric and postmenopausal periods. *Clin Obstet Gynecol* 20:113–122.

23. Wild, R. A., et al. 1987. Declining adrenal androgens: an association with bone loss in aging women. *Proc Soc Exp Biol Med* 186:355–360.

24. Rozenberg, S., et al. 1990. Age, steroids and bone mineral content. *Maturitas* 12:137–143.

25. Nordin, B. E. C., et al. 1985. The relation between calcium absorption, serum dehydroepiandrosterone, and vertebral mineral density in postmenopausal women. *J Clin Endocrinol Metab* 60:651–657.

26. Sambrook, P. N., et al. 1988. Sex hormone status and osteoporosis in postmenopausal women with rheumatoid arthritis. *Arthritis Rheum* 31:973–978.

27. Ibid. *Note:* Administration of adrenal corticosteroids suppresses ACTH secretion by the pituitary gland, which results in reduced secretion of a number of adrenal hormones.

28. Browne, E. S., et al. 1992. Dehydroepiandrosterone: Antiglucocorticoid action in mice. *Am J Med Sci* 303:366–371.

29. Crilly, R. G., D. H. Marshall, and B. E. C. Nordin. 1979. Metabolic effects of

corticosteroid therapy in post-menopausal women. *J Steroid Biochem* 11:429–433.

30. Devogelaer, J. P., J. Crabbe, and C. N. De Deuxchaisnes. 1987. Bone mineral density in Addison's disease: Evidence for an effect of adrenal androgens on bone mass. *Br Med J* 294:798–800.

31. Hollo, I., et al. 1977. Osteopenia. *Ann Intern Med* 86:637.

32. Mortola, and Yen, 696–704.

33. Northrup, C. Personal communication.

17

Do Food Allergies
Contribute to Osteoporosis?

We all know someone who has experienced an allergic reaction to a food or a food additive. Some of us have suffered such reactions ourselves. Foods such as peanuts, shellfish, or strawberries, and additives such as tartrazine (yellow dye #5) or sulfites may cause severe asthma, swelling, skin rashes, or other symptoms in susceptible individuals. These types of immediate allergic reactions are quite obvious and are easy to recognize.

MASKED FOOD ALLERGY

Less obvious, and more controversial, are the hidden or "masked" allergies. These types of allergies are more difficult to identify, both because they are often delayed (sometimes for as long as several days after ingestion of an offending food) and because they do not occur every time the food is eaten. Recognition of masked allergies is also hampered by the fact that many of the symptoms are not generally thought to be related to allergies. Nevertheless, doctors who have taken a serious look at masked food allergy have found it to be one of the most common causes of symptoms. According to James Breneman, M.D., past president of the food allergy division of the American Academy of Allergy, food allergy is the cause of up to 60% of all symptoms that are inadequately diagnosed and treated by a typical family doctor.[1]

Problems that can be caused by food allergy are numerous and diverse, and include fatigue, anxiety, depression, insomnia, food cravings, recurrent infections, chronic nasal congestion, irritable bowel syndrome (spastic colon), inflammatory bowel disease (ulcerative colitis or Crohn's disease), eczema, canker sores, chronic hives, muscle aches, arthritis, migraines and other headaches, asthma, frequent urination, bedwetting, and infantile colic. Food allergy is even responsible in some cases for cardiovascular problems, including high blood pressure, angina, and heart rhythm disturbances. Obviously, food allergy is not the only cause of these many symptoms, but it is one of the most common causes and is probably the one most frequently overlooked.

DIAGNOSING FOOD ALLERGY

Food allergy should be suspected in individuals who have a childhood history of infantile colic, recurrent ear infections, sore throats, runny nose, "growing pains," asthma, eczema, or "getting sick all the time." Since allergy is hereditary, people who have a family history of allergy are more likely to be allergic themselves. Certain signs on a physical examination may also suggest that allergies are present. Many allergic individuals have *allergic shiners,* a term used to describe the puffy, dark circles under the eyes similar to the way your eyes look when you have not gotten enough sleep. Allergy may also cause edema (swelling) of the face, lower legs, or other areas of the body.

Skin tests are notoriously unreliable for detecting masked food allergy. Blood tests (such as the radioallergosorbent test, or RAST) that measure antibodies against specific foods are somewhat more accurate, but even these tests have a high rate of error. Probably the most reliable (and certainly the least expensive) method of identifying hidden food allergies is to do an *elimination diet* for several weeks.

Elimination Diets

A typical elimination diet is one that completely prohibits all foods containing sugar, wheat, dairy products, corn products, eggs, citrus fruits, coffee, tea, alcohol, and all food additives. If your chronic symptoms disappear or improve considerably while you are on the diet, then you are probably allergic to one or more of the foods you have eliminated. In addition, by following such a diet for several weeks, you will have "unwaterlogged" your system and "unmasked" your allergies. With your body in this hyperalert state, reintroducing foods to which you are allergic will provoke rapid and exaggerated reactions—usually the same symptoms that had ceased with the diet.

Using the elimination diet followed by individual food testing, I have been able to help thousands of patients rid themselves of problems that had often plagued them for years—problems for which they had spent thousands of dollars on medical bills in an unsuccessful search for relief. One of the elimination diets I use in my practice is presented in Appendix B. This diet is a modification of "Elimination Diet A" from the book *Tracking Down Hidden Food Allergies*, by William G. Crook, M.D.[2] Although some people have been able to follow this diet on their own, I recommend professional supervision to make sure that you follow the program properly and that you do not develop any nutritional deficiencies.

DO FOOD ALLERGIES PROMOTE OSTEOPOROSIS?

For many people who have suffered from asthma, migraine headaches, bowel problems, arthritis, or any of the other conditions listed previously, the chance to be free from these troubling problems is reason enough to stay away from allergenic foods. However, there is also reason to believe that proper attention to food allergy might reduce your likelihood of developing osteoporosis. As discussed in Chapter 2, bones are living tissue, just like the brain, the heart, the respiratory system, the joints, and the skin. It seems improbable that allergy, which affects so many different tissues and organs in the body, would not also affect the bones.

Continual ingestion of allergenic foods can cause subtle or overt damage to the gastrointestinal tract, resulting in malabsorption and deficiencies of a wide range of nutrients. As I pointed out in previous chapters, deficiencies of one or more of a long list of vitamins and minerals can increase the risk of developing osteoporosis. Although a cause and effect relationship between food allergy and osteoporosis has not been proven several factors point to a possible association, including the relationship between osteoporosis and celiac disease, and the effect of allergy on nutrient absorption, nutritional deficiencies, and certain hormones.

Celiac Disease

A classic example of a food allergic condition associated with bone loss is *celiac disease,* an intestinal disorder caused by intolerance to the gluten grains: wheat, oats, barley, and rye. The most common manifestations of celiac disease are persistent diarrhea, bloating, and abdominal pain. In people with celiac disease, the gluten grains act like a bulldozer to the small intestine, ripping away the billions of microscopic folds that make up the normal absorptive surface, and replacing them with a flattened, poorly functioning mucosa (mucous membrane). Consequently, individuals with celiac disease usually suffer from multiple nutritional deficiencies. However, after they eliminate the gluten grains from their diet, both nutrient absorption and overall nutritional status improve.

Osteoporosis and Celiac Disease

Osteoporosis is known to occur frequently in people with celiac disease. Studies show that bone loss is not a result of the disease itself but is, rather, a consequence of eating the foods to which the individual is intolerant. Nicoletta Molteni, M.D., and associates at the

University of Milano, in Milano, Italy, recently compared bone mineral density in patients with celiac disease to that of healthy people who were the same age (control group).[3] In adults who had only recently been diagnosed and who had not, therefore, been consuming a gluten-free diet, bone mineral density was significantly lower than in the control group. However, bone mineral density was similar between the control group and celiac patients who had been following a gluten-free diet since childhood. These findings demonstrate that celiac patients who consume the foods to which they are intolerant have an increased risk of developing osteoporosis, whereas avoiding these foods eliminates the excess risk.

A recent study showed that a gluten-free diet can also reverse established osteoporosis in celiac patients. In a group of children with celiac disease, bone mineral density of the radius (a bone in the forearm) was significantly lower than in healthy children. However, when these patients followed a gluten-free diet for an average of about fifteen months their bones exhibited "catch-up" growth; that is, their bone density increased at a greater rate than that of the healthy children.[4]

Allergic Malabsorption: A Common Condition?

It is important to note that many individuals with celiac disease do not have the characteristic severe diarrhea and intestinal malabsorption that doctors associate with this condition. In fact, in the Italian study 9 of the 29 patients studied had no gastrointestinal symptoms at all, but only iron-deficiency anemia as a presenting complaint. An additional five patients had chronic gastrointestinal symptoms that had previously been misdiagnosed as irritable bowel syndrome or spastic colon.

The discovery of celiac disease in patients who do not have the classic symptoms suggests that celiac disease, or at least subtle variations of this condition, may be more common than is generally believed. Doctors do not typically recommend biopsies of the small intestine unless a patient has severe and persistent gastrointestinal symptoms. Therefore, we do not know how often the typical flattened small-intestinal mucosa found in celiac disease is present in people with other diseases. One study, however, suggested that gluten-induced small bowel damage is not limited to people with obvious celiac disease. When the healthy relatives of individuals with celiac disease were fed a normal diet supplemented with 40 g/day of gluten, significant damage occurred in the mucosa of the jejunum (a portion of the small intestine). These same gluten-induced intestinal abnormalities were also seen in four patients with altered immune function who ingested gluten.[5]

Thus, it is possible that a substantial proportion of the population might develop intestinal abnormalities resulting in nutrient malabsorption if they ingest large quantities of wheat, corn, or other gluten grains to which they are allergic. Furthermore, the potential effect of food intolerance on nutritional status is not limited to gluten grains. Studies in children who are allergic to milk, soy, or egg have demonstrated severe intestinal damage following ingestion of the offending food. It is likely that allergenic foods cause similar, though perhaps less severe, problems in the intestinal tract of adults.

Allergy and Nutritional Deficiency

The relationship between allergy and nutritional deficiency has been documented in several other studies. Among a group of 330 patients with recurrent aphthous ulcers (canker sores in the mouth), a condition frequently caused by food allergy, 14.2% were deficient in iron, folic acid, vitamin B12, or a combination of these nutrients.[6] Other disorders related to food allergy have also been associated with nutritional deficiencies. For example, magnesium deficiency is frequently encountered in people with migraines, asthma, or inflammatory bowel disease; vitamin B6 deficiency is common in asthma and rheumatoid arthritis; and low levels of zinc are often seen with eczema, rheumatoid arthritis, and aphthous ulcers. In a study of 46 children with food allergies, 67% had rough or dry skin (suggesting deficiencies of essential fatty acids or vitamin A), compared to only

9% of nonallergic children.[7] In another study comparing 150 allergic children and 102 healthy children, poor growth was frequently associated with allergy. Control of the allergies was commonly followed by a growth spurt.[8]

In summary, these studies suggest that nutritional deficiencies are likely to occur in individuals with food allergies, possibly as a result of nutrient malabsorption. Since deficiencies of various nutrients may promote osteoporosis, allergy control represents another potentially beneficial strategy in the battle against bone loss.

Allergy and Hormones

Allergies may lead to bone loss by affecting certain hormones. One of the body's natural defenses against allergic reactions is to secrete corticosteroids (cortisonelike molecules) from the adrenal glands. Indeed, the standard medical treatment for acute allergic reactions is prednisone or other corticosteroids. But, one of the major side effects of prednisone therapy is osteoporosis. It is also known that Cushing's syndrome, a disorder characterized by excessive secretion of adrenal corticosteroids, causes osteoporosis. It is quite possible, then, that a continual outpouring of corticosteroids in response to repeated allergic reactions might also cause osteoporosis.

Allergy also apparently impairs the body's ability to utilize testosterone, a hormone known to build bone.[9] The combined effects of excess corticosteroid secretion and impaired utilization of testosterone may be important factors contributing to bone loss.

CONCLUSION

Identifying and avoiding allergenic foods is one of the major components of nutritional therapy. Millions of Americans suffer from chronic complaints caused by food intolerance. Although the evidence is circumstantial, it appears that avoiding allergenic foods may provide the added benefit of reducing osteoporosis risk.

NOTES

1. Breneman, J. C. 1978. *Basics of food allergy.* Springfield, Ill.: C. C. Thomas.
2. Crook, W. G. 1980. *Tracking down hidden food allergies.* Jackson, Tenn.: Professional Books.
3. Molteni, N., et al. 1990. Bone mineral density in adult celiac patients and the effect of gluten-free diet from childhood. *Am J Gastroenterol* 85:51–53.
4. Mora, S., et al. 1993. Effect of gluten-free diet on bone mineral content in growing patients with celiac disease. *Am J Clin Nutr* 57:224–228.
5. Doherty, M., and R. E. Barry. 1981. Gluten-induced mucosal changes in subjects without overt small-bowel disease. *Lancet* 1:517–520.
6. Wray, D., et al. 1978. Nutritional deficiencies in recurrent aphthae. *J Oral Pathol* 7:418–423.
7. Cardi, E., et al. 1988. Roughness of skin in food allergy. *Lancet* 1:886.
8. Cohen, M. B., and L. E. Abram. 1948. Growth patterns of allergic children. *J Allergy* 19:165–171.
9. Green, J. R. B., et al. 1977. Reversible insensitivity to androgens in men with untreated gluten enteropathy. *Lancet* 1:280–282.

18

You Are What You Assimilate

Everyone has heard the saying, "You are what you eat." But, from the standpoint of nutritional biochemistry, it would be more accurate to say "You are what you assimilate." For some people, eating wholesome foods high in vitamins and minerals is still not enough to maintain good nutritional status. If the nutrients present in your food are not effectively transported from your intestinal tract into your bloodstream, you can develop nutritional deficiencies despite a supposedly adequate diet. Digestion and absorption are extremely complex processes, and the efficiency of these processes can vary greatly from person to person.

Numerous reports in medical journals have demonstrated that nutrients can often be used to treat various medical conditions. In practice, however, while nutrient therapy may work very well for one person, the same treatment may have little or no effect on another individual with the same medical problem. Similarly, some people who do not respond to nutrients taken by mouth will improve significantly if the nutrients are given by injection. These observations suggest that some individuals do not assimilate nutrients properly from their diet, and that measures to enhance their digestive and absorptive capabilities might have a beneficial effect on their health.

In previous chapters, I presented evidence that at least fourteen different nutrients play a role in maintaining bone mass and preventing osteoporosis. I recommended various high-nutrient foods and nutritional supplements to insure that you obtain enough of what your bones need. However, what you put in your mouth may not necessarily be what ends up in your system. It is, therefore, important to discuss some of the factors involved in proper nutrient assimilation.

THE IMPORTANCE OF CHEWING

Nutritional science is a complicated subject, requiring an understanding of biochemistry, physiology, and clinical medicine. But, some of the basic principles of good nutrition are rather obvious. In our zeal to provide the most up-to-date, sophisticated recommendations we sometimes forget to emphasize the obvious—like the importance of chewing. One of the most important elements of good eating is to chew thoroughly. There is great truth in the Upton Sinclair statement that "Nature will castigate those who don't masticate." Nature has endowed you with teeth for a very important reason: to chew your food.

One of the effects of chewing is to mix your food with saliva, which contains important digestive enzymes. Chewing also reduces the size of food particles, thereby increasing the surface area upon which the digestive juices can act. As food passes through the gastrointestinal tract, there is only a limited time during which digestion and absorption take place. The smaller the particles that come into contact with digestive juices, the more efficient the digestive process will be. That point can be illustrated by an analogy.

Imagine that your digestive tract is a large vat filled with warm water and that the food to be digested is fifty pounds of ice. If the ice is in the form of a single fifty-pound block, then it might take the better part of a day for it to be "digested" (melted) by the warm water. If, on the other hand, the ice is crushed prior to being placed in the water it will melt completely in a matter of minutes or even seconds. Similarly, food chewed thoroughly has a better chance of being digested than food swallowed whole. Even the strongest digestive system on the planet would have a difficult time dealing with a meal that has been "wolfed down" on the run.

It is surprising how often I encounter patients who are doing (almost) everything they can to stay well. They eschew junk food, get plenty of sleep and exercise, avoid caffeine and alcohol, and maintain a positive attitude toward life. And yet, for them, eating is done at a pace only a half-step slower than inhaling. Many such individuals complain of chronic digestive problems such as intestinal bloating, belching, flatulence, constipation, or diarrhea. They come to me seeking expert advice on how to alleviate their "irritable bowel syndrome." In some cases, the only expert advice they need to hear is to chew each mouthful forty times.

YOU NEED STOMACH ACID

One of the other major factors that influences nutrient absorption is stomach secretions. Gastric juice contains, among other things, a protein-digesting enzyme called *pepsin* and a vitamin B12-binding substance known as *intrinsic factor*. In addition, a healthy stomach is capable of secreting *hydrochloric acid* at a concentration so strong that it could corrode a copper penny.

Acidity is measured in units called *pH*. The lower the pH, the more acidic the solution. The pH scale is logarithmic, which means that a one-point drop in pH is equivalent to a tenfold increase in acidity, and a two point drop is equivalent to a one hundredfold increase. The normal pH of stomach juice is about 1.5, compared to about 7.4 for blood. What that means is that stomach secretions are nearly one million times more acidic than blood. Producing such a highly concentrated acid requires an enormous amount of metabolic energy, and one must assume that nature has a good reason for endowing the stomach with such extraordinary acidifying capability.

Activates Pepsin

Gastric acid serves three major functions. First, it activates the enzyme pepsin, which depends on an acidic environment to function normally. As a proteolytic (protein-digesting) enzyme, pepsin breaks down the structural proteins within foods, thereby allowing the release of vitamins, minerals, and other nutrients into the "digestive soup" where they can be absorbed into the bloodstream. If there is not enough acid to promote efficient peptic digestion, then a significant proportion of the vitamins and minerals will remain bound up within food particles and unavailable for absorption.

Increases Nutrient Solubility

A second important function of gastric acid is to increase the solubility of nutrients after they have been released from a food or a nutritional supplement. For most nutrients to be absorbed across the intestinal wall into the bloodstream, they must first be dissolved or put into solution. Some food components, such as sugar or salt, dissolve easily in water or in other nonacidic solutions. However, some vitamins and minerals are only weakly soluble, except in acidic solutions. Calcium carbonate, for example, one of the forms of calcium commonly used in nutritional supplements, dissolves easily in a dilute hydrochloric acid solution, but dissolves hardly at all in water. It seems, therefore, that a well-functioning stomach is required for certain nutrients to be absorbed.

Barrier against Infection

A third function of gastric acid is as a protective barrier against microorganisms from the outside world. Bacteria, viruses, and fungi inhaled or ingested would normally be destroyed by the strong acid secreted by the stomach. As a result, the stomach and small bowel are normally sterile—that is, free of microorganisms. Individuals who lack stomach acid, on the other hand, are frequently found to have any number of different organisms growing in their stomach or small intestine. One can only guess what effect this overgrowth of organisms might have on the rest of the body. Abnormal intestinal organisms might conceivably interfere with the absorption of nutrients. In addition, colonization of the bowel by abnormal microbes may cause a shift in the normal intestinal flora. Doctors who routinely perform stool cultures on their patients find that what grows in the stool is often quite different from what the textbook calls normal bacterial flora. Some of these abnormal bowel bacteria may result from overuse of antibiotics, which tend to destroy the normal intestinal bacteria. However, some of this problem may be due to hypochlorhydria (discussed next) and may, therefore, be correctable with hydrochloric acid supplementation.

It is important to remember that much of the vitamin K obtained by the body is synthesized by normal intestinal bacteria. If the wrong bacteria are living in your gastrointestinal tract then you may be at risk for vitamin K deficiency. As pointed out in Chapter 3, vitamin K plays an important role in osteoporosis prevention and fracture healing, and vitamin K deficiency may be common in people with osteoporosis.

LOW STOMACH ACID

With all of the advertisements we see on television for antacids to neutralize "excess stomach acid," it might seem hard to believe that too little acid may be as big a problem as too much. However, studies have shown that *hypochlorhydria* (the medical term for inadequate secretion of gastric hydrochloric acid) is a relatively common occurrence, particularly among the elderly. According to one medical text, approximately 10 to 15% of the general population has hypochlorhydria. Among individuals over the age of sixty, the prevalence of hypochlorhydria may be as high as 50%. A number of medical conditions are also associated with low stomach acidity, such as asthma; allergies; rosacea (a type of acne); vitiligo (a skin condition); thyroid disorders (both hyperthyroidism and hypothyroidism); gallbladder disease; and various rheumatologic conditions including rheumatoid arthritis, systemic lupus erythematosus, and Sjogren's syndrome.

Symptoms of Hypochlorhydria

Individuals with hypochlorhydria frequently experience various gastrointestinal symptoms. One of the most common is bloating after meals. The type of bloating that is due to low stomach acid typically begins near the end of a meal or up to thirty minutes later. Food allergy may also cause intestinal bloating and is sometimes difficult to distinguish from hypochlorhydria, in terms of time of onset. Bloating due to insufficient pancreatic secretions is also fairly common, but typically develops an hour or more after a meal. People with low stomach acid also experience a sensation of food sitting in their stomach, almost like a piece of lead. This sensation is most likely to occur after ingestion of beef or other high-protein foods. Hypochlorhydria may also cause constipation or, less often, diarrhea, particularly morning diarrhea. On the other hand, some individuals with hypochlorhydria have no abdominal complaints at all.

Physical signs suggestive of low stomach acid include weak or brittle fingernails, prominent capillaries around the nose and cheeks, and hair loss in women. The hair loss may be due to iron deficiency, since iron absorption requires hydrochloric acid and iron deficiency is known to be associated with hair loss. When appropriate therapy with hydrochloric acid is given the gastrointestinal symptoms and physical signs often disappear.

Hydrochloric Acid and Nutrient Absorption

The relationship between gastric acidity and intestinal calcium absorption has been looked at in a number of studies. In one such study, the stomachs of rats were exposed to radiation in order to induce hypochlorhydria. These rats absorbed less calcium from the diet and had lower bone mineral content than control rats which had normal stomachs.[1] Studies in humans have also demonstrated the importance of gastric acid on calcium absorption. Most of these investigations have shown that hypochlorhydria reduced the absorption of calcium.[2,3] Although not all studies have confirmed these findings,[4,5] it appears that hydrochloric acid is required, at least in some circumstances, for calcium to be absorbed efficiently.

Other studies have shown that absorption of folic acid also depends on the presence of adequate hydrochloric acid.[6] It has further been reported that absorption of copper, iron, and chromium require hydrochloric acid. Other nutrients, such as zinc, manganese, and magnesium, may depend on hydrochloric acid for absorption, but that possibility has not yet been studied.

STOMACH ACID AND OSTEOPOROSIS

To review what we have learned so far, hypochlorhydria may result in reduced absorption of calcium, copper, folic acid, and other nutrients related to osteoporosis prevention. Hypochlorhydria is also relatively common in the elderly, the same age group most susceptible to developing osteoporosis. Even in younger individuals, an association between osteoporosis and low stomach acid has been shown. In one study, seventy-nine people between the ages of 16 and 53 underwent gastric analysis. Those who had evidence of alveolar bone loss (the bone that supports the teeth) produced less than half as much hydrochloric acid as those without alveolar bone loss.[7]

MEASURING GASTRIC ACIDITY

Several laboratory tests may provide indirect information about gastric acidity. Analysis of the hair of individuals with hypochlorhydria often reveals a majority of the minerals to be below the normal range. In addition, the finding of undigested meat fibers in a microscopic analysis of the stool suggests that there is not enough hydrochloric acid to break down protein completely. Although these tests are suggestive, they do not provide a clear picture of stomach function. The most reliable method of assessing gastric acidity is called *gastric analysis by radiotelemetry.* In this test the patient swallows a small capsule, containing a pH-measuring device and a radiotransmitter. The capsule measures the gastric pH and transmits this information to a machine, which prints out a continuous reading of the gastric acidity. Several times during the test the patient is given 2 teaspoons of a solution of baking soda. The time required for the stomach to neutralize the baking soda and to reacidify the gastric contents is considered a measure of the acidifying capability of the stomach. While this test is performed by many nutrition-oriented practitioners, it is relatively unknown among the general medical community. In fact, the average doctor rarely considers the possibility that low stomach acid could be a factor in health and disease.

A gastric analysis may be worthwhile for individuals with osteoporosis, particularly those who have some of the signs, symptoms, associated medical conditions, and laboratory abnormalities discussed. If hypochlorhydria is identified supplementation with hydrochloric acid may be worthwhile. Unfortunately, not everyone is in a position to have such a test either because it is not available locally or because of the cost and inconvenience. In some instances, a therapeutic trial with hydrochloric acid under medical supervision may be warranted.

HYDROCHLORIC ACID THERAPY

Hydrochloric acid is usually given as a supplement in the form of either betaine hydrochloride or glutamic acid hydrochloride. Some of these supplements also contain pepsin. Capsules are preferable to tablets because people with a weak stomach may not be able to break down a tablet completely, allowing the tablet to sit in the stomach and cause heartburn. The usual trial dosage is 10 to 30 grains (10 grains equals about 600 mg) of betaine hydrochloride or glutamic acid hydrochloride per meal, taken preferably with the first few bites of the meal. Individuals with proven hypochlorhydria may sometimes need more than that. Side effects such as heartburn occur occasionally and may require a reduction in dosage. Individuals taking aspirin, ibuprofen, or other nonsteroidal anti-inflammatory drugs should not take hydrochloric acid, because the combination may increase the risk of developing a peptic ulcer.

In many instances, hydrochloric acid therapy not only relieves gastrointestinal symptoms but also enhances overall health by improving nutritional status. Symptoms such as weak fingernails and hair loss may also improve. By increasing the absorption of bone-building nutrients, hydrochloric acid may help prevent osteoporosis in people with hypochlorhydria. However, because of the potential for side effects hydrochloric acid therapy should be supervised by a health practitioner.

PANCREATIC ENZYMES

Another important contributor to the digestive process is the pancreas. Enzymes secreted by the pancreas into the gastrointestinal tract facilitate the digestion of protein, carbohydrates, and fat. A weakness of the pancreas may result in malabsorption of vitamin D, vitamin K, and zinc, all of which are related to bone health. Severe pancreatic insufficiency may result from chronic alcoholism or chronic pancreatitis. Symptoms and signs of mild pancreatic enzyme deficiency include bloating after meals (usually occurring an hour or so after the end of the meal), oily or foul smelling stools (due to the presence of excessive amounts of fat in the stool), and dry, flaky skin (resulting from poor absorption of essential fatty acids and vitamin A). Supplementing the diet with pancreatic enzymes may be beneficial. Bromelain (from pineapple stem) or papain (from papaya) may be effective substitutes for pancreatic enzymes.

An occasional individual is unable to produce enough bile salts, which are required for absorption of essential fatty acids and vitamins A, D, E, and K. Administering bile salts may be beneficial for these individuals. In the interest of safety, pancreatic enzymes and bile salts should be used only under medical supervision.

CONCLUSION

This chapter has presented information on ways of promoting better nutrient absorption. Insuring proper absorption of vitamins and minerals is an essential component of an osteoporosis-prevention program. Although supplementation with digestive aids is relatively safe, it is not entirely risk-free. It is therefore advisable that you seek appropriate professional advice before experimenting with digestive supplements.

NOTES

1. Mahoney, A. W., and D. G. Hendricks. 1974. Role of gastric acid in the utilization of dietary calcium by the rat. *Nutr Metabol* 16:375–382.
2. Hunt, J. N., Johnson, C. 1983. Relation between gastric secretion of acid and urinary excretion of calcium after oral supplements of calcium. *Dig Dis Sci* 28:417–421.
3. Recker, R. R. 1985. Calcium absorption and achlorhydria. *N Engl J. Med* 313:70–73.
4. Knox, T. A., et al. 1991. Calcium absorption in elderly subjects on high- and low-fiber diets: Effect of gastric acidity. *Am J Clin Nutr* 53:1480–1486.
5. Bo-Linn, G. W., et al. 1984. An evaluation of the importance of gastric acid secretion in the absorption of dietary calcium. *J Clin Invest* 73:640–647.
6. Russell, R. M., S. D. Krasinski, and I. M. Samloff. 1984. Correction of impaired folic acid (Pte Glu) absorption by orally administered HCl in subjects with gastric atrophy. *Am J Clin Nutr* 39:656.
7. Brechner, J., and W. D. Armstrong. 1941. Relation of gastric acidity to alveolar bone resorption. *Proc Soc Exp Biol Med* 48:98–100.

19

Aluminum and Osteoporosis

As we have stated previously, osteoporosis is becoming increasingly prevalent. While pathologists of the nineteenth century knew of the existence of fragile and porous bones, these phenomena were considered more of a medical curiosity than a common problem. It was not until after World War I that osteoporosis came to be recognized as a prevalent condition. Furthermore, between around 1950 and 1980, the incidence of osteoporotic fractures (adjusted for the age of the population) has doubled in various parts of the world. While our sedentary existence has probably contributed to the rise in osteoporotic fractures, osteoporosis also develops in many physically active individuals.

A great deal of circumstantial evidence suggests that pollution of our environment with various toxic chemicals is a contributing factor to the causation of many of the "diseases of Western civilization," including heart disease, diabetes, cancer, liver and kidney diseases, and autoimmune disorders. If one considers that osteoporosis is also a disease of modern civilization, then the possibility exists that pollution plays a role in the development of bone loss, as well. As bone is living tissue that constantly exchanges fluids, nutrients, and chemicals with the rest of the body, it is unlikely that bone tissue would escape the effects of toxins that are damaging other parts of the body.

ALUMINUM IS EVERYWHERE

Of all the thousands of chemicals that man has introduced into the environment during the past century, aluminum is perhaps the most ubiquitous. Aluminum is the metal of the modern world. It is a major component of buildings, automobiles, furniture, and appliances. It is used to wrap foods and is the most commonly used metal in soft drink and beer cans. Aluminum is also present as an additive in a wide range of foods and is added to some municipal water supplies to remove particulate matter. Aluminum is also a major ingredient in many antacids.

Human beings have no known nutritional requirement for aluminum and, under certain circumstances, it is clearly toxic. This toxicity has been most evident in individuals with chronic renal (kidney) failure whose kidneys are too impaired to excrete aluminum efficiently. In the 1970s, before doctors were aware of the threat of aluminum poisoning, some dialysis centers were using aluminum-containing tap water to dialyze their kidney patients. The buildup of aluminum in these patients caused a condition, dialysis encephalopathy, characterized by confusion, neurologic abnormalities, seizures, coma, and even death. The incidence of dialysis encephalopathy decreased dramatically after doctors began using aluminum-free solutions for dialysis. Aluminum bone disease, manifesting as bone pain, fractures, and muscle weakness, has also been reported in individuals with renal failure.

ACCUMULATION IN BODY TISSUES

There is disagreement about whether aluminum exposure can cause disease in people whose kidneys function normally. It has been generally assumed that only a small fraction of ingested aluminum is actually absorbed into the bloodstream, and that the aluminum that does make it into the body is efficiently excreted from the body through the urine. However, newer evidence suggests that this assumption may be incorrect—that aluminum can, indeed, accumulate in the body, even when the kidneys are perfectly healthy.

In one study, twenty patients scheduled for brain surgery were given antacids for ten days prior to the operation, to prevent stress ulcers. Twenty-four other patients were given antacids for four weeks prior to undergoing a diagnostic bone biopsy. One of the antacids used was rich in aluminum (Maalox 70), while the other contained very little aluminum (Riopan). Brain and bone tissues obtained during the procedures were analyzed for aluminum. In patients receiving the high-aluminum antacid (Maalox 70), the concentrations of aluminum in brain and bone tissue were elevated. In contrast, aluminum levels were normal in the tissues of patients given the low-aluminum antacid.[1] This study clearly demonstrates that orally ingested aluminum is absorbed into the body and is deposited in our tissues.

RELATIONSHIP TO ALZHEIMER'S DISEASE

The fact that ingested aluminum can migrate to the brain should heighten our concerns about the proposed relationship between aluminum and Alzheimer's disease. This type of dementia has apparently become more common in recent times. Aluminum concentrations in the brain of individuals with Alzheimer's disease have been found to be fifteen times higher than those in people dying of other causes. While it is possible that aluminum accumulates in the brain as a consequence, rather than as a cause, of this condition, animal studies suggest the opposite is really the case. When rats are fed aluminum in their diet, they develop an abnormality of their brain cells called *neurofibrillary tangles,* the same abnormality seen in the brain of those with Alzheimer's disease.

THE OSTEOPOROSIS CONNECTION

The fact that ingested aluminum can also end up in bones has important implications for osteoporosis. The accumulation of aluminum in bone appears to reduce the formation of osteoid (areas of new bone formation), while at the same time increasing the amount of bone resorption.[2] The result of this dual action of aluminum would be to accelerate bone loss.

Individuals who habitually consume aluminum-containing antacids to relieve gastrointestinal symptoms may be consuming large amounts of this toxic metal. Some antacids contain more than 200 mg of aluminum per tablet. Ingestion of ten of these tablets per day would expose the user to 100 to 200 times the average daily aluminum intake of 10 to 20 mg. At least some of the aluminum contained in antacids is absorbed, as demonstrated by an increase in the urinary excretion of aluminum following ingestion.[3] Recent investigations in humans have shown that even small doses of aluminum-containing antacids can substantially increase urinary calcium excretion.[4] The effect is even greater when the dosage of antacids is larger, but increasing the dietary intake of calcium partially prevents the adverse effects of antacids. However, aluminum also appears to have other adverse effects on calcium metabolism and on bone itself.

In 1960, a syndrome of severe bone pain, osteomalacia (softening of the bones), and pseudofractures developed in some people who had been consuming aluminum hydroxide–containing antacids for prolonged periods of time.[5] One of the effects of aluminum is to bind phosphorus in the intestinal tract, thereby inhibiting its absorption. Phosphorus depletion is one of the causes of aluminum-induced bone loss because phosphorus is an essential component of bone crystals. Osteoporosis has also been reported to occur in rabbits that were fed aluminum sulfate.[6] In a study in rats, administering aluminum by injection increased the amount of bone resorption and reduced the formation of new bone.[7]

SOURCES OF ALUMINUM EXPOSURE

If the aluminum present in antacids can damage our bones, then we should also be wary of the countless other sources of absorbable aluminum in our lives. No one can say for sure whether our daily exposure to aluminum plays an important role or only an insignificant one with respect to osteoporosis. Some of you will choose to live your life as you always have, without worrying too much about another substance only *suspected* of being a problem. Others may want to do everything possible (hopefully, short of becoming neurotic or bankrupt) to avoid ingesting a potentially toxic substance such as aluminum. Whatever your philosophy of life, awareness of the main sources of aluminum will help you make more informed choices.

Beverage Cans

One of the most frequently encountered sources of aluminum is beverage cans. Supposedly, the thin lacquer coating on the inside walls of the can prevents aluminum from being dissolved by the contents of the can. However, imperfections in this coating might allow contact between the aluminum and the liquid, causing some of the aluminum to dissolve. In a study of fifty-two beverages obtained from Australia, New Zealand, and Thailand, the aluminum content of noncola soft drinks in cans was six times higher than that of the same drinks in bottles.[8] The aluminum concentration of cola drinks was nearly three times greater in cans than in bottles. These differences were not seen for beers, probably because soft drinks are more acidic than beers and are therefore capable of dissolving more aluminum. The soft drinks in aluminum cans contained up to 3.9 mg of aluminum per can, a substantial amount, considering that dissolved aluminum is probably more efficiently absorbed than are various solid forms of aluminum. It would seem, therefore, that one important way to reduce your exposure to absorbable aluminum would be to purchase your drinks in glass bottles, rather than in aluminum cans.

Cookware

Another significant source of this toxic metal is aluminum cookware. When foods are heated in aluminum pots and pans, some of the aluminum is leached into the food. The amount of aluminum dissolved increases with higher cooking temperatures and with longer periods of cooking. Acidic foods such as tomato sauce leach aluminum to a much greater extent than do neutral or alkaline foods. However, even pure water can do a job on an aluminum pot. Whereas the concentration of aluminum in tap water was 22 mcg/l, the concentration increased by seventy-fivefold to a level of 1,640 mcg/l after the water was heated in an aluminum pot.[9] That level is more than thirty times the recommended water quality limit of 50 mcg/l. Aluminum cookware is preferred by some people because of its light weight and because it transmits heat efficiently. However, these advantages are outweighed by the potential harm from increased aluminum intake. Aluminum cookware cannot, therefore, be recommended under any circumstance. Stainless steel, glass, or other appropriate cooking vessels are preferable. It should be noted, however, that pots and pans that have an aluminum underside and a stainless steel cooking surface are safe to use.

Tap Water

As mentioned previously, aluminum is added to some municipal water supplies to help remove particulate matter from the water. If you drink such water, you are receiving a gratuitous dose of poison every time you turn on the tap. Although the overall concentration of aluminum in city water may be small, the amount of water you drink is probably relatively large. Consequently, the amount of aluminum derived from drinking water can add up.

Other concerns have been voiced about the safety of municipal water. Chlorine, used to kill bacteria, is a powerful oxidizing agent, which has the potential to cause damage to your cells and tissues. Some scientists believe that chlorination of the water supply promotes heart disease and cancer and that there are safer ways (such as using ozone) of keeping our water free of dangerous organisms.

In addition, there is some evidence that fluoridated water can cause allergic reactions and may increase the risk of cancer. With the newer tooth-bonding techniques available to dentists, ingesting fluoridated water may no longer be necessary to prevent cavities.

The logical response to being faced with a water supply polluted with aluminum, chlorine, fluoride and all of the industrial chemicals emanating from the factories upstream is to use bottled water (from a reputable company) for drinking and cooking, or to purchase a filter that removes the unwanted materials from your tap water. Because filtering or distilling water removes most of the essential trace minerals, people who drink filtered or distilled water should probably supplement their diet with a broad-spectrum multiple-mineral tablet.

Food Additives

A number of additives found in our food supply also contain aluminum. For example, sodium aluminum phosphate is used to release carbon dioxide gas from baking soda to leaven self-rising cake mixes, pancake batters, and frozen doughs. Aluminum phosphates are also used as emulsifying agents in processed American cheeses. Baking powder is also a significant source of aluminum. Other aluminum compounds, known as alums, are used as firming agents in pickled vegetables and maraschino cherries. Processed cheese contains about 50 mg of aluminum per slice; a medium-sized pickled cucumber contains 5 to 10 mg. Certain buffered aspirins and other prescription or over-the-counter drugs also contain aluminum. In general, whole (unprocessed) foods are low in aluminum, whereas some processed foods contain substantial amounts of the metal. Nutritionists recommend whole foods anyway because of their higher nutrient content. Reducing your exposure to aluminum and other food additives is yet another reason to eat the "natural" way.

By making some basic changes in the type of food, water, and medications you consume and in the cookware and underarm deodorants you use (many such deodorants also contain aluminum), you can substantially reduce the amount of aluminum that gets into your body. However, regardless of how hard you try, it is impossible to avoid this metal completely.

CITRATE PROMOTES ALUMINUM ABSORPTION

It is important, therefore, that you be aware of one substance that can increase the absorption and toxicity of aluminum. That substance is citrate or, when present in its acidic form, citric acid. Studies have shown that citrate binds tightly to aluminum, forming aluminum citrate. This particular form of aluminum is exceptionally well absorbed from the intestinal tract into the bloodstream. When aluminum and citrate are present at the same time in the gastrointestinal tract, aluminum citrate will form and increase the absorption of aluminum.

The consequences of ingesting these compounds simultaneously can be serious for people with renal failure. One woman who was given citrate (for the treatment of a condition called acidosis) along with an aluminum-containing antacid developed severe aluminum toxicity, resulting in brain damage and death.[10] In people with normal renal function who can excrete most of the aluminum that is absorbed, the outcome would not be so serious.

Nevertheless, repeated ingestion of aluminum and citrate could increase the body burden of aluminum, potentially resulting in damage to the brain, the bones, or other tissues. In one study, when healthy volunteers ingested 1.6 grams of aluminum (hydroxide), the urinary excretion of aluminum over the following twenty-four hours increased by 45 mcg. However, when citrate was ingested along with the aluminum, the twenty-four-hour urinary aluminum excretion increased more than sevenfold to 327 mcg, suggesting that more aluminum had been absorbed.[11] Other studies also confirm an interaction between these two compounds.[12] Rats fed aluminum citrate had higher aluminum concentrations in the brain and bones than rats fed aluminum hydroxide. Administering lemon juice (which is high in citric acid) to healthy men increased aluminum levels in the blood serum to a greater extent than ingestion of either substance alone.

Several possible situations might find you ingesting aluminum and citrate simultaneously. If you took an antacid or a buffered aspirin along with orange juice or another citrus fruit (grapefruit, lemon, or lime), you would ingest this combination. If you took an aluminum-containing antacid for your stomach and followed it with magnesium citrate (a laxative), you would form a large amount of aluminum citrate in your gastrointestinal tract. Certain nutritional supplements contain minerals that are complexed with citrate; calcium citrate, for example, is preferred by some people because it is thought to be absorbed more efficiently than other calcium salts. Some products also contain zinc citrate or magnesium citrate. If you use aluminum-containing antacids, be sure not to consume citrus fruits or minerals complexed with citrate at the same time.

GETTING RID OF ANTACID DEPENDENCE

Having discussed the potential dangers of aluminum-containing antacids throughout this chapter, it should by now be obvious that if you must take an antacid, you should choose one that is low-aluminum or aluminum-free. High-aluminum antacids include Maalox, ALternaGEL, Amphojel, Basaljel, and Mylanta. Riopan contains a moderate amount of aluminum. Alka Seltzer and Tums contain little or no aluminum.

Making Nutritional Changes

Of course, where antacids are concerned, the best solution is to eliminate the need for the medication in the first place. Millions of Americans who depend on antacids to treat peptic ulcers or preulcer conditions of the stomach or duodenum could probably find a successful alternative in nutritional and natural medicine. The first advice I give to patients who have ulcers, indigestion, or dyspepsia is to chew their food slowly and thoroughly and to avoid refined sugar, white flour, fried foods, caffeine, and alcohol. Avoidance of tobacco products is also recommended, although quitting cigarettes is usually much more difficult than making dietary changes.

Fortunately, the new nicotine patches have increased the success rate of individuals trying to stop smoking. Herbal products that contain an extract of oat straw (Avena sativa) have also been shown to reduce the craving for cigarettes.[13]

A significant proportion of people who make these changes find that their stomach problems clear up and they no longer need to take antacids. Of those who do not improve, many have allergies or intolerances to specific foods, such as dairy products, wheat, corn, or eggs. Food allergy or intolerance can be identified by going on an elimination diet for about three weeks (see Chapter 17 and Appendix B). If the symptoms (heartburn, bloating, nausea, and so on) disappear during that time, then reintroducing one at a time the foods that have been removed from the diet generally provokes reactions. Avoiding those identified as the offending foods controls the symptoms.

More than half of the patients I have seen who "cleaned up" their diet and searched for specific food intolerances have been able to control their chronic gastrointestinal symptoms. Of those who had depended on antacids to make it through the day, nearly all were able to discontinue them without having a recurrence of their symptoms.

When Diet Changes Fail

When dietary modifications alone do not produce satisfactory results, a simple extract of licorice root (known as deglycyrrhizinated licorice, DGL) frequently comes to the rescue. DGL has been shown to be as effective as the widely used antiulcer drugs Tagamet and Zantac as a treatment for peptic ulcer.[14] Clinical experience suggests that it is also frequently effective for much of the heartburn and indigestion for which people take antacids. Although whole licorice root works just as well, the whole root contains a substance called glycyrrhizin, which has corticosteroid activity and can therefore cause adverse side effects. Fortunately, scientists have determined that the glycyrrhizin can be removed from licorice root without losing the antiulcer and intestinal healing effects of licorice. Deglycyrrhizinated licorice, so named because 97% of the glycyrrhizin has been removed, is sold in Europe as an antiulcer drug and is available in health food stores in the United States. DGL is generally well tolerated and does not cause cortisonelike side effects. However, in people who are taking corticosteroids by mouth, there is a small chance that DGL might increase both the effectiveness and the toxicity of these medications. On rare occasions, DGL causes loose bowels in susceptible individuals.

SUMMARY

This chapter has presented evidence that exposure to aluminum from numerous sources in our environment is one of the factors that promotes the development of osteoporosis. Although this relationship has not been proven, it is possible that the increasing proliferation of aluminum-containing products is one reason that the age-adjusted incidence of osteoporotic fractures has doubled during the past thirty years. Suggestions are presented for minimizing your exposure to this metal and preventing excessive amounts of aluminum from being absorbed into your system.

NOTES

1. Anonymous. 1986. Aluminum in antacids shown to accumulate in brain and bone tissue. *Gastroenterol Observer* 5(6):1–2.

2. Kaehny, W. D. 1985. Newer understanding of aluminum metabolism. *IM* 6(6):131–140.

3. Walker, J. A., R. A. Sherman, and R. P. Cody. 1990. The effect of oral bases on enteral aluminum absorption. *Arch Intern Med* 150:2037–2039.

4. Spencer, H., and L. Kramer. 1983. Antacid-induced calcium loss. *Arch Intern Med* 143:657–659.

5. Spencer, H., et al. 1982. Effect of small doses of aluminum-containing antacids on calcium and phosphorus metabolism. *Am J Clin Nutr* 36:32–40.

6. Anonymous. 1982. Food, pots, processing agents and antacids—all are sources. *Med Tribune,* 28 April, 12.

7. Goodman, W. G., J. Gilligan, and R. Horst. 1984. Short-term aluminum admin-

istration to the rat. Effects on bone formation and relationship to renal osteo-malacia. *J Clin Invest* 73:171–181.

8. Gerrans, C. 1992. Soft drinks tend to boost aluminum intake. *Med Tribune,* 23 July, 17.

9. Jackson, J. A., H. D. Riordan, and C. M. Poling. 1989. Aluminium from a coffee pot. *Lancet* 1:781–782.

10. Kirschbaum, B. B., and A. C. Schoolwerth. 1989. Acute aluminum toxicity associated with oral citrate and aluminum-containing antacids. *Am J Med Sci* 297:9–11.

11. Walker, Sherman, and Cody, 2037–2039.

12. Ibid.

13. Anand, C. L. 1971. Effect of Avena sativa on cigarette smoking. *Nature* 233:496.

14. Glick, L. 1982. Deglycyrrhizinated liquorice for peptic ulcer. *Lancet* 2:817.

20

Other Heavy Metals: Lead, Cadmium, and Tin

In Chapter 19, we discussed the relationship between aluminum and osteoporosis. In this chapter, we will investigate the possibility that three other toxic metals—lead, cadmium, and tin—also play a role in the development of bone loss. Each of these metals is used extensively in industry and is present in our food, our water, and elsewhere in the environment.

LEAD

Lead poisoning has long been recognized as an important public health problem in the United States. Because it is one of the most widely used industrial metals, there are many ways in which we can become exposed to lead. While lead has no known biological function in the body, it is capable of accumulating in our tissues and causing a wide range of toxic effects. Furthermore, the more we learn about this metal, the more dangerous it looks. Levels of exposure once considered safe are now known to cause adverse effects on the brain and nervous system.

Low-level lead poisoning can cause vague symptoms such as muscle aches, fatigue, irritability, lethargy, joint pains, trouble concentrating, headaches, vomiting, and weight loss. More severe lead poisoning can cause brain damage, gastrointestinal complaints, and neuritis. Lead is also thought to be a factor in high blood pressure, heart disease, and stroke.

Sources of Lead Exposure

It is hard to get away from lead in our modern society. With advances in civilization, our exposure to lead has increased geometrically. Worldwide production of lead was only about 100,000 tons 300 years ago. By 1930, that figure had increased tenfold to one million tons per year. In 1980, worldwide production was three million tons.[1] Approximately 200,000 tons of industrial lead aerosols are emitted annually into the atmosphere of the Northern Hemisphere. The air in cities in North America contains 500 to 10,000 ng of lead per cubic meter. Tiny particles of lead present in the air are inhaled and absorbed through the lungs. Much of this airborne lead eventually falls to the ground, where it is incorporated into the soil and enters the food chain.

Even though our exposure to lead has been reduced in recent years as a result of the ban on leaded gasoline, there are still many important sources of exposure. According to a recent report by the Environmental Protection Agency, the drinking water in 130 cities, including Boston, New York, Philadelphia, Washington, Seattle, San Francisco, and Phoenix, contains excessive amounts of lead.[2] Sampling of 660 large public water supplies revealed that about 32 million Americans drink water that exceeds the federal safety standard of 15 parts per billion (ppb). In 10 cities, lead was above 70 ppb, with Charleston, South Carolina, having the worst reading, 211 ppb.

The solubility of lead increases markedly at water pH of 6.8 or less.[3] This pH is only very slightly acidic; some municipal water supplies have a pH of 6.0 or less. At that pH, significant amounts of lead may leach from pipes. Municipal water systems have consequently begun treating the water supply with lime or other chemicals to decrease its acidity, in an attempt to reduce the amount of lead that corrodes from pipes and solder.

Canned foods are another significant source of lead. Of 256 products in metal cans examined for lead, 62% contained 100 mcg/l or more, 37% contained 200 mcg/l or more, and 12% contained 400 mcg/l or more. Of products in glass containers, only 1% had more than 200 mcg/l of lead.[4] Some individuals, including plumbers, glass manufacturers, printers, plastics or battery manufacturers, and construction workers, may be exposed to excessive amounts of lead on the job. Other sources of lead include some paints, ceramic ware, and some cosmetics.

Because of our ubiquitous exposure to this toxic metal, it has been suggested that our entire society suffers from subtle lead poisoning. It is difficult to test this hypothesis, since virtually everyone has accumulated at least some lead in their tissues. In one study, the concentration of lead in the skeletons of Americans was found to be 500 times higher than that in the bones of Peruvians who lived in an unpolluted environment 1800 years ago.[5] It has been further estimated that the content of lead in our diet is 100 times greater than in the diet of prehistoric peoples.

Lead and Osteoporosis

Several studies have shown that lead poisoning can cause abnormalities in the bones, including osteoporosis. According to a report by the Environmental Protection Agency, nine individuals, ages 15 to 22, suffering from chronic lead poisoning had X-ray evidence of bone abnormalities, including radio-opaque bands in growing bones, diffuse osteoporosis, and vertebral malformations.[6] In another study, injection of lead salts into animals caused the appearance of large numbers of osteoclasts (the cells that cause bone resorption) and resorption of bone in all parts of the skeleton.[7] The degree of lead exposure in these studies was considerably greater than the amount the average person is exposed to. However, we cannot rule out the possibility that a lifetime of low-level lead exposure is one of the factors contributing to the epidemic of osteoporosis in industrialized societies.

It is noteworthy that lead does interfere with the hormone progesterone. In one study, administering 0.5% lead in the diet of pregnant mice prevented the rise in plasma progesterone that normally occurs during pregnancy.[8] As discussed in Chapter 15, progesterone plays an important role in maintaining bone mass. Progesterone deficiency may be quite common, as indicated by the number of women with premenstrual syndrome, habitual miscarriages, and osteoporosis who have reportedly responded to progesterone therapy. It is possible that low-level lead exposure is one of the factors that promotes progesterone deficiency.

Lead and Nutrient Interactions

The relationship between nutritional status and susceptibility to lead poisoning has been extensively studied, both in animals and humans. It is well documented that deficiencies of calcium, magnesium, zinc, vitamin C, iron, and certain B-vitamins increases the toxic effects of lead. Conversely, correcting these deficiencies reduces lead toxicity. In some cases, supplementing with vitamins and minerals beyond the amounts required to correct a deficiency has been shown to reduce lead toxicity even further. Most of the nutrients listed here have been shown to protect against osteoporosis. Perhaps one of the effects of these nutrients is to minimize the bone-resorbing effect of lead.

Avoiding Lead Exposure

There are a few simple measures you can take to minimize your exposure to lead. Have your tap water analyzed for lead. If the concentration is above the accepted limit, you should consider drinking and cooking with bottled water. If that is not feasible, then run the tap at least one full minute before using the water. Most of the lead found in tap water accumulates while the water is sitting in the pipes for a long period of time. Running the tap for awhile flushes all of the "old" water out of the pipes; the water that follows will contain substantially less lead. Another simple change you can make is to avoid canned foods and to emphasize instead fresh food and food packaged in glass. If you live near a major highway or an industrial plant, you should not grow your own vegetables because the soil around your house may contain too much lead. It may also be wise to supplement your diet with moderate doses of the vitamins and minerals listed previously, as an additional insurance policy against lead exposure. One possible exception is iron supplementation. Although some people are iron deficient, others have a tendency to accumulate excessive amounts of iron. These individuals may actually increase their risk of developing heart disease and diabetes if they take iron unnecessarily. A simple test called a *serum ferritin level* can be ordered by your doctor to determine whether taking iron is appropriate for you.

CADMIUM

Cadmium is used in the manufacturing of batteries, plastics, paints, textiles, and fertilizers. Both metal and plastic water pipes contain some cadmium and this mineral is present in food and water. Some "organic" fertilizers used by home gardeners are made from sewage sludge, which contains large amounts of cadmium. When cadmium is deposited in the soil it remains there for a long time; more than 99% stays within one yard of the soil surface over a ten-year period. Cadmium in the soil is taken up by grains and vegetables and is ultimately ingested by humans. Cadmium is a significant component of cigarette smoke and is efficiently absorbed by the lungs into the bloodstream. Other significant sources of cadmium include motor oil, tires, and galvanized parts of motor vehicles.

Cadmium and Bones

Workers exposed to excessive levels of cadmium may develop high blood pressure and kidney disease. Cadmium toxicity may also adversely affect the bones. During World War II, a mysterious condition, the "ouch-ouch disease," afflicted many individuals living along the banks of the Jintsu River in Japan. Eventually traced to cadmium toxicity, the symptoms included bone pain, severe osteomalacia (softening of the bones), and multiple pathologic fractures.[9] Other studies have also found an association between cadmium exposure and bone disease. Among a group of coppersmiths who were chronically exposed to cadmium fumes, 18.5% had a highly significant increase in urinary calcium excretion.[10] Rats fed 10, 50, or 100 parts per million of cadmium in their diet had bone abnormalities reminiscent of osteomalacia. These abnormalities were increasingly more severe with increasing concentrations of cadmium in the diet.[11]

To what extent cadmium exposure contributes to osteoporosis is unknown. However, the association between cigarette smoking and bone loss may be due, at least in part, to the high concentration of cadmium found in tobacco smoke. Because cadmium is more efficiently absorbed through the lungs than through the gastrointestinal tract, smoking is probably one of the most significant sources of cadmium for the average individual. The possibilty that secondhand smoke could affect the bones of nonsmokers should also be kept in mind.

Cadmium and Nutrient Interactions

Aside from avoiding cigarettes and choosing to live and work far away from polluting factories, there is not much you can do to avoid cadmium exposure. However, there is evidence that the level of certain vitamins and minerals in your diet may influence your susceptibility to cadmium toxicity. The effects of individual nutrients on cadmium toxicity and tissue accumulation of cadmium have been extensively studied in animals. While the damaging effects of cadmium were generally worse in nutrient-deficient animals, nutrient supplements partially counteracted the toxic effects of this mineral. Nutrients that have been shown to interact with cadmium include calcium, zinc, iron, copper, vitamin B6, vitamin C, and selenium.[12,13]

The interaction between cadmium and zinc has been further demonstrated on bone tissue. In one study, minute quantities of cadmium stimulated the resorption of mouse bone in the test tube. However, this effect was prevented by the addition of zinc.[14]

It is interesting to note that most of the vitamins and minerals that prevent the accumulation and toxicity of cadmium have been shown elsewhere in this book to protect against osteoporosis. While each of these nutrients has a wide range of effects in the body, it is possible that one of the ways in which they preserve bone mass is to minimize the adverse effects of cadmium exposure.

TIN

Even though tin has been recognized as an essential nutrient since the 1960s, its exact function in the body is not understood. However, because of our widespread exposure to tin as an industrial pollutant and because of the ability of tin from cans to leach into the food, the possibility of toxicity from tin is a far greater concern than the risk of a nutritional deficiency of this trace element.

The sources of tin exposure are many. Stannous chloride (the term *stannous* refers to tin) is a tin salt frequently used as a chemical preservative. Stannous fluoride is present in some toothpastes as a source of fluoride. Tin compounds are components of some fungicides and insecticides, and they are also used as stabilizers in some packaging materials. Small amounts of tin from these sources enter the food supply. Tin is also an atmospheric pollutant, arising from its use in industry, and can enter the body through the lungs.

Perhaps the most significant source of tin is food and beverage containers. The usual daily intake of tin among people who consume only fresh, frozen, and bottled foods is about 3 mg. Foods packed in cans that are totally coated with lacquer usually contain only a very small amount of tin, not enough to increase the daily intake significantly. However, some foods, such as citrus juices, pineapple juice, and applesauce, are often packed in uncoated cans. The tin content of the foods taken from these cans has been found to be as high as 10 to 35 mg per cup. The amount of tin in these foods increases further if the foods are stored for several months at temperatures greater than 40°C (a temperature that would easily occur in a warehouse during the summer). The concentration of tin may also increase quite a bit if the food is stored in the can after it has been opened. In one study, storing food in an opened can in the refrigerator increased the tin level to 100 mg per cup.[15] The corrosion of tin is more rapid with acidic foods than with neutral or alkaline foods. In addition, citric acid (or citrate), which binds to tin, can cause an enormous amount of tin corrosion.[16]

Toxicity due to ingestion of tin has been reported in animals. Rats fed 0.3% tin in their diet had growth retardation, anemia, and structural changes in the cells of the liver. These effects were reduced by feeding them additional copper and iron, suggesting that some of the toxic effects of tin may result from interference with other essential nutrients.[17] Chronic administration of tin to animals has also caused impaired immune system function, and reduced tissue levels of zinc, copper, and calcium. In a study of human volunteers, administering 36 mg of tin (from stannous chloride), an amount easily obtainable from one or two helpings of a canned food, inhibited the absorption of zinc.[18]

Tin and Osteoporosis

Tin is known to accumulate in bone in proportion to the amount in the diet. Because excess tin has been shown to damage other tissues in the body, its presence in bone could have an adverse effect there, as well. In one study, rats were fed tin at concentrations of 10, 50, 100, or 250 parts per million (ppm) in the diet. At tin concentrations of 50 ppm or greater, blood levels of calcium were reduced and the calcium content of certain areas of the femur bone was diminished.[19] These changes were not seen with 10 ppm of tin. However, a concentration of 50 ppm or more of tin would not be difficult to achieve from a diet that contained some canned foods, particularly if those foods were stored for long periods of time in a hot environment or if the cans were left open in the refrigerator for several days.

Tin may affect bones either through direct toxicity or indirectly, through an interaction between tin and certain essential nutrients. As mentioned, exposure to tin may increase the requirement for zinc and copper, both of which play a role in bone metabolism and osteoporosis.

Another potentially harmful effect of tin is to inhibit the production of gastric hydrochloric acid. This strong acid, normally secreted by the stomach, appears to be necessary for digestion and absorption of many different nutrients including calcium, copper, and folic acid (see Chapter 18). Each of these nutrients is involved in maintaining strong bones. By reducing the amount of gastric acid produced, tin might promote a deficiency of these important nutrients.

Avoiding Exposure

The amount of tin many of us are ingesting from tin cans and other sources may be sufficient to have an adverse influence on bone health. The simplest and possibly the most effective measure to take to reduce your exposure to this metal is to purchase foods in glass, rather than in tin containers. If you must use food from cans, do not store the cans for long periods of time or at high temperatures. After you open the can store the unused contents in a glass or plastic container. Although it has not been proven, there is some evidence that supplementing your diet with zinc and copper may help minimize the effects of tin exposure. Iron supplementation may also be beneficial. However, as mentioned, you should have your serum ferritin level measured before taking iron supplements.

HOW DANGEROUS ARE HEAVY METALS?

Although aluminum, lead, cadmium, and tin are clearly toxic at high doses, are the levels we are exposed to day by day really a cause for concern? Unfortunately, we cannot answer that question with any degree of certainty. Neither, however, can we be sure that these levels of exposure are perfectly safe. It is possible that the subtle

effects of these metals on bone and other tissues that occur gradually over time may be undetectable in short-term laboratory studies
using animals.

Two factors might lead scientists to underestimate the adverse
effects of persistent low-level exposure. First, when a toxic substance is studied in the laboratory, the animals are not simultaneously exposed to the thousands of other poisons that humans face
every day in the real world. Many foreign chemicals are detoxified
in the body by the same mechanisms. The presence of many different chemicals might overwhelm these defense mechanisms. As
a result, a small amount of a single chemical that is tolerated by rats
in a controlled environment might cause damage to humans living
in a polluted world.

Second, laboratory animals are usually fed diets of exceptionally high nutritional quality. The vitamin and mineral content of
these diets often greatly exceeds that of human diets, particularly
ones that contain large amounts of sugar, white flour, processed
foods, and oils. Deficiencies of calcium, zinc, copper, manganese,
vitamin C, and other nutrients are known to aggravate the effects of
heavy metal exposure. Consequently, the adverse effects of these
metals on marginally nourished humans may be underestimated if
one studies only exceptionally well-nourished animals. Thus, the
dangers of heavy metal exposure to human health may be greater
than laboratory studies suggest.

NOTES

1. Settle, D. M., and C. C. Patterson. 1980. Lead in Albacore: Guide to lead pollution in Americans. *Science* 207:1167–1176.
2. Gutfeld, R. 1992. Excessive lead found in water of many cities. *Wall Street
   Journal,* 21 October, B7.
3. Pocock, S. J. 1980. Factors influencing household water lead: A British national
   survey. *Arch Environ Health* 35:45–51.
4. Mitchell, D. G., and K. M. Aldous. 1974. Lead content of foodstuffs. *Environ
   Health Perspect* 7:59.
5. Settle and Patterson, 1167–1176.
6. Mongelli Sciannameo, N. 1972. Radiologic observations on the skeletal appa-

ratus of young persons affected by chronic lead poisoning. In *Biological aspects of lead: An annotated bibliography,* edited by I. R. Campbell and E. G. Mergard, Abstract 1355 (May):260. Washington D.C.: US Environmental Protection Agency.

7. Hancox, N. 1956. The osteoclast. In *The biochemistry and physiology of bone,* edited by G. H. Bourne, 234. New York: Academic Press.

8. Jacquet, P., et al. 1977. Plasma hormone levels in normal and lead-treated pregnant mice. *Experientia* 33:1375–1377.

9. Anonymous. 1971. "Ouch-Ouch" disease: Due to cadmium. *JAMA* 216:154.

10. Scott, R., et al. 1978. Hypercalciuria related to cadmium exposure. *Urology* 11:462–465.

11. Takashima, M., S. Moriwaki, and Y. Itokawa. 1980. Osteomalacic change induced by long-term administration of cadmium to rats. *Toxicol Appl Pharmacol* 54:223–228.

12. Fox, M. R. S. 1983. Cadmium bioavailability. *Fed Proc* 42:1726–1729.

13. Pond, W. G., and E. F., Walker, Jr. 1975. Effect of dietary Ca and Cd level of pregnant rats on reproduction and on dam and progeny tissue mineral concentrations. *Proc Soc Exp Biol Med* 148:665–668.

14. Suzuki, Y., et al. 1990. Preventive effect of zinc against cadmium-induced bone resorption. *Toxicology* 62:27–34.

15. Greger, J. L. 1984. Newer understanding of tin metabolism. *IM* 5(4):173–178.

16. Nagy, S., R. Rouseff, and S-V. Ting. 1980. Effects of temperature and storage on the iron and tin contents of commercially canned single-strength orange juice. *J Agric Food Chem* 28:1166–1169.

17. Pfeiffer, C. C. 1978. *Zinc and other micronutrients.* New Canaan: Keats, 134–135.

18. Valberg, L. S., P. R. Flanagan, and M. J. Chamberlain. 1984. Effects of iron, tin, and copper on zinc absorption in humans. *Am J Clin Nutr* 40:536–541.

19. Yamaguchi, M., K. Sugii, and S. Okada. 1981. Inorganic tin in the diet affects the femur in rats. *Toxicol Lett* 9:207–209.

21

Does Acid Rain Damage Your Bones?

I have suggested previously that certain aspects of environmental pollution may be responsible in part for the increasing prevalence of osteoporosis in some industrialized nations. Toxic metals such as aluminum, lead, cadmium, and tin were mentioned as pollutants that might cause bone loss. Contamination of our food, water, and air with hydrazine compounds might, by interfering with vitamin B6 metabolism, also contribute to the development of osteoporosis. It is likely that of the hundreds of thousands of other chemicals modern man is exposed to, at least some will be found to have an adverse effect on our bones.

ACID RAIN

One factor usually overlooked that may significantly affect bone health is acid rain. In some parts of the world, rain is no longer a source of fresh water providing nourishment to plant and animal life. Rather, it has become a source of deadly acid, capable of causing damage to all living beings. The acidity of rain is due primarily to the release of acidic sulfur and nitrogen compounds during the burning of sulfur-rich coal. These compounds are oxidized in the atmosphere to form sulfuric acid and nitric acid, both highly potent acids.

Rainwater is normally mildly acidic (pH 5.6) because some of the carbon dioxide present in the atmosphere dissolves in rain to form carbonic acid. Acid rain is defined as rainwater with a pH below 5.6. The pH of rain in areas susceptible to acid rain is often between 4.1 and 4.7, more than ten times as acidic as normal rainwater. Values less than 4.1 have also been reported. The world record of less than 2.0 was achieved during one long rainfall in West Virginia in 1978. That value represents a degree of acidity more than 5,000 times greater than that of "healthy" rainwater. During the past thirty years, there has been a substantial increase in acid precipitation, primarily a result of increasing use of sulfur-rich coal.

Damage to Ecosystems

Severe degradation of some ecosystems due to acid rain has already been reported in the United States, Canada, Scotland, Norway, Sweden, and other parts of Europe. The loss of fish, as well as other animal and vegetable life, has been attributed to acid rain. Although no clear proof has yet emerged concerning the toxic effects of acid rain on humans, it would be surprising if it were not causing at least subtle damage to our health.

ACID RAIN AND OSTEOPOROSIS

Excessively acidic rain could promote osteoporosis in two ways. First, by increasing the acidity of our drinking water, acid rain might put increased stress on our internal buffering mechanisms. Calcium is one of the major buffers against acid. When the body is exposed to excess acidity, calcium is released from the bones to buffer the acid, thereby preventing a dangerous fall in blood pH. It is quite possible that continual exposure to acidic water would cause excessive leaching of calcium from our bones. A second way in which acid rain could damage our bones is by promoting the release of toxic metals, such as aluminum, lead, and cadmium from rocks and soil. Acid rain can increase human exposure to lead not only by leaching it from rocks and soil, but also by lowering the pH of tap water, which would tend to dissolve more lead from the plumbing. Acid rain also corrodes exterior surfaces. On surfaces covered with lead-based paint or aluminum siding, acid rain would tend to dissolve these metals into the water.

One study has shown that these potential adverse effects of acid rain are more than just theoretical.[1] In areas of the northeastern United States, an association between the acidity of rainwater and the concentration of dissolved aluminum in surface and ground water was demonstrated. The excess aluminum in high-acid areas was derived primarily from weathering of rock. The aluminum concentration in acidified lakes in the Adirondacks was 10 to 50 times higher than concentrations in neutral waters from the same region. Soils exposed to acid rain also had high concentrations of dissolved aluminum. These findings suggest that acid rain may increase aluminum levels in both streams and lakes, which would ultimately increase the concentration of aluminum in the food chain. The possibility that exposure to aluminum is one of the causes of osteoporosis was discussed in Chapter 19.

Environmentalists have been concerned for a long time about the effects of acid rain on our environment. Most of the concerns have been over the destruction of aquatic life, particularly in lakes. Some have suggested that the progressive deforestation of areas of Europe is being caused by acid rain. It has also been observed that pied flycatchers breeding close to acidified lakes and therefore feeding on insects contaminated with aluminum had defective mineralization of their eggshells.[2] Will we eventually discover that exposure to acid precipitation also causes defective mineralization of our bones?

REDUCING OUR EXPOSURE

Acid rain can be controlled in two major ways. One way is to remove the offending compounds from high-sulfur coal before the coal is burned. We already possess the technology to produce cleaner-burning coal, although such coal is somewhat more expensive. The other alternative is to switch to low-sulfur coals entirely. Certainly, attempts to achieve greater energy efficiency and to seek cleaner sources of energy such as solar power would also have a positive impact. As a society, we must decide whether the benefits to our health and our planet outweigh the economic costs of making these changes.

NOTES

1. Cronan, C. S., and C. L. Schofield. 1979. Aluminum leaching response to acid precipitation: Effects on high-elevation watersheds in the Northeast. *Science* 204:304–306.
2. Mjoberg, B. 1989. Aluminium-induced hip fractures: A hypothesis. *J Bone Joint Surg* 71B:538–539.

Additional Suggested Reading

Anonymous. 1984. Acid rain: Toxic metals. *Lancet* 1:659–660.
Anonymous. 1985. Acid-rain and human health. *Lancet* 1:616–618.

22

Exercise and Osteoporosis

It has long been known that bones develop in a way that resists the forces acting upon them. This means that repeated application of a physical stress to a bone will actually cause that bone to remodel and become stronger. For example, in a study of eighty-four professional tennis players, X rays showed that the humerus (a bone in the upper arm) on the playing side was thicker than the same bone in the other arm.[1]

Conversely, immobilization and weightlessness result in accelerated bone loss. A rapid increase in urinary calcium excretion has been observed in astronauts during their time in space. In addition, in a group of patients who had been placed on strict bed rest because of low back pain, bone mineral content of the lumbar spine decreased at an astounding 0.9% per week. Attempts to prevent this rapid bone loss through diet, nutritional supplements, or drugs have not been successful. Thus, physical activity plays a crucial role in maintaining bone mass.

SEDENTARY LIFESTYLES

As mentioned earlier, the age-specific incidence of osteoporotic fractures has doubled over the past thirty years or so. I have suggested that nutritional deficiencies and environmental pollutants may have contributed to this increasing incidence of fractures. However, it is also likely that a reduction in physical activity is involved. We live in an age where nearly everyone has an automobile, several television sets, and dozens of electrical appliances designed to decrease their work around the house. The amount of physical activity required to perform the essential tasks of living is now substantially less than it was in generations past. Surveys have shown that some individuals lie around watching television as much as 6 to 8 hours per day. The "couch potato" appears to be primarily a phenomenon of the past several decades. Nowadays, even most jobs have us sitting at desks, instead of doing physical labor as in past generations.

EXERCISE STRENGTHENS BONES

A number of studies have shown that a person's bone mass is directly related to the amount of physical exercise that individual does. For example, an international survey of hip fractures in women from various countries showed an age-adjusted incidence (per 100,000 women) from as high as 146 in Sweden, to 62 in England, to as low as 7.5 in South African Bantu. These differences could not be explained by hormonal status or by dietary calcium intake, but were related to the degree of physical activity undertaken by the different populations.[2] In another study of 46 postmenopausal women, those who were physically fit had greater bone mineral content in the femur and the lumbar spine than did women of the same age who were less fit.[3] The relationship between bone mass and exercise was also investigated in a group of 41 male and female long-distance runners, ages 50 to 72. Compared to an age-matched group of sedentary individuals, both male and female runners had approximately 40% more bone mineral content (measured by CT scan of the first lumbar vertebra).[4]

It has also been clearly demonstrated that women who engage in exercise programs can either prevent or reverse postmenopausal bone loss. Forty-eight postmenopausal women were randomized to a control group, aerobic exercise, or aerobic exercise plus strengthening exercises. The aerobic exercises, done three times a week for one year, consisted of 5 to 10 minutes of stretching and calisthenics, followed by thirty minutes of walking, jogging, and various dance routines. The strength-training group had an additional 10 to 15 minute session of isometric and isotonic contractions of various muscle groups in the limbs and trunk, using free weights attached to the wrists and ankles. After one year, both exercise groups had significantly greater bone mass than the control group. The women who did strengthening exercises had greater bone mass than those who did aerobic exercises alone, but the difference was not statistically significant.[5]

The beneficial effects of exercise do not appear to be limited by age, and may be realized even in the very elderly. Twelve women with an average age of eighty-four years participated in an exercise program thirty minutes a day, three days a week for three years, while eighteen women of similar age served as controls. The exercises included walking and running in place, knee lifts, toe touches, arm lifts, and more than eighty-five other movements. After three years, the women participating in physical activity had an average increase in bone mass at the distal radius (a bone in the forearm) of 2.29%, compared to an average loss of 3.28% in the control group.[6]

Weight Bearing Exercise versus Swimming

The bone-building effect of exercise is due mainly to the repetitive physical stress applied to the bone. It is therefore generally believed that only weight-bearing exercises are capable of increasing bone density. A *weight-bearing* exercise is one in which pressure is placed on a bone either by the weight of the body or by the force of muscular contraction. Exercises that fall into this category include

walking, running, jumping on a trampoline, playing tennis or basketball, and weight lifting.

Most people have assumed that an exercise such as swimming,
although good for the cardiovascular system, would not increase
bone density. That is because the arm and leg motions involved in
pulling oneself through the water do not exert a large amount of
force on the bones. However, recent findings suggest that swimming may also increase bone density. Male competitive swimmers,
ages 40 to 83, who did not participate in other forms of regular
exercise had significantly greater bone mass at the forearm and in
the vertebrae than did nonathletes. In a similar study of thirty-seven
older female swimmers, there was a trend toward increased vertebral bone density compared to nonathletes (130 vs. 109 mg/ml),
but the difference did not quite reach statistical significance.[7] These
results indicate that, while swimming does not increase bone density as much as weight-bearing exercises, it does have a beneficial
effect on bone mass. That finding is important, because some elderly individuals with osteoporosis are too frail to perform weight-
bearing exercises. For them, swimming can be a gentle, nontrau-
matic way to increase their bone mass.

For younger and more robust individuals, weight-bearing exercises may be preferable because they are more effective at building and maintaining bone mass. However, intense exercises such as
running and weight lifting also carry a greater risk of injury, and the
potential benefits must be weighed against the risks. The choice of
what type of exercise to do should be made on an individual basis,
perhaps in consultation with a doctor or physical trainer.

What is most important is that you engage in some type of
regular exercise, perhaps thirty minutes at a time, three or four times
a week. To promote optimal health, exercise should be started early
in life and continued into your later years. Not only does exercise
improve bone mass, but it has also been shown to be associated
with a lower risk of heart disease, diabetes, cancer, high blood
pressure, fatigue, depression, anxiety, insomnia, and other common
problems. When my sedentary patients begin an exercise program
they almost always begin to feel better in many ways within a month
or two.

OVERDOSING ON EXERCISE

One possible downside to exercise has been reported in female long-distance runners who develop amenorrhea (loss of menstruation). In one study of twenty-eight long-distance runners, bone mineral density of the lumbar spine was signficantly lower in those with amenorrhea than in runners whose menstrual periods remained normal.[8] This reduction in bone mass was apparently related more to amenorrhea than it was to excessive exercise. Another group of nine amenorrheic women with reduced bone mineral density were observed over a fifteen-month period. In the two women who remained amenorrheic there was a further 3.4% loss of bone mineral density. However, in the seven women in whom menstruation resumed there was a 6.3% increase in bone mass.[9]

Even though amenorrhea, rather than exercise per se, appears to be the cause of bone loss in long-distance runners, a reduction in the amount of exercise for sufferers may be beneficial. In one study, seven female runners with exercise-induced amenorrhea and decreased vertebral bone mineral density were reevaluated after fifteen months. In four runners who took calcium supplements and reduced their weekly running distance by 43%, there was a 5% increase in average body weight, a return of menstruation, and a 6.7% increase in average bone mineral density. Three runners who did not change their running distance had no change in body weight and continued to have amenorrhea. Although all three women took calcium supplements, there was no change in bone mineral density.[10] These studies indicate that women who develop amenorrhea as a result of long-distance running are at increased risk for bone loss. However, if menstruation returns either spontaneously or as a result of reducing the amount of running, then bone mass will be restored.

Diet and Amenorrhea

There may also be some dietary factors that predispose some women to exercise-induced amenorrhea. In a study of female distance runners, some with amenorrhea and some with normal menstrual cycles, calcium intake and percentage of body fat were similar between the two groups. However, those with amenorrhea ingested significantly fewer calories and less protein than did those with normal menstruation. Among those with amenorrhea, 82% consumed less than the Recommended Dietary Allowance for protein. The authors of the study concluded that abnormal eating patterns are associated with amenorrhea and bone loss in female runners.[11] Athletes who stop menstruating should therefore consider reducing their total amount of exercise and should make sure to consume a diet that provides adequate amounts of calories, protein, vitamins, and minerals.

NOTES

1. Sinaki, M. 1988. Exercise and physical therapy. In *Osteoporosis: Etiology, diagnosis, and management,* edited by B. L. Riggs and L. J. Melton, III, Chapter 19. New York: Raven Press.

2. Chalmers, J., and K. C. Ho. 1970. Geographical variations in senile osteoporosis. The association with physical activity. *J Bone Joint Surg* 52B:667–675.

3. Pocock, N. A., et al. 1986. Physical fitness is a major determinant of femoral neck and lumbar spine bone mineral density. *J Clin Invest* 78:618–621.

4. Lane, N. E., et al. 1986. Long-distance running, bone density, and osteoarthritis. *JAMA* 255:1147–1151.

5. Chow, R., J. E. Harrison, and C. Notarius. 1987. Effect of two randomised exercise programmes on bone mass of healthy postmenopausal women. *Br Med J* 295:1441–1444.

6. Smith, E. L. 1982. Exercise for prevention of osteoporosis: A review. *The Physician and Sportsmedicine* 10(3):72–82.

7. DeBenedette, V. 1987. Study: Swimming may increase bone density. *The Physician and Sportsmedicine* 15(12):49.

8. Nelson, M. E., et al. 1986. Diet and bone status in amenorrheic runners. *Am J Clin Nutr* 43:910–916.

9. Drinkwater, B. L., et al. 1986. Bone mineral density after resumption of menses in amenorrheic athletes. *JAMA* 256:380–382.

10. Lindberg, J. S., et al. 1987. Increased vertebral bone mineral in response to reduced exercise in amenorrheic runners. *West Med J* 146:39–42.

11. Nelson, et al. 910–916.

23

Does Thyroid Hormone Cause Osteoporosis?

During the past five years, several studies have been published suggesting that treatment with thyroid hormones accelerates bone loss. These reports have alarmed the medical community, causing doctors to reduce the dose of thyroid hormone in some patients, or to forego treatment altogether. Because of these reports, millions of Americans who are receiving thyroid hormones to treat an underactive thyroid gland or to shrink a thyroid nodule are living in fear that their medical treatment is slowly eroding their bones.

The possible connection between thyroid hormone treatment and osteoporosis was of particular concern to practitioners of nutritional medicine. Many of us are followers of the late Broda Barnes, M.D., author of the landmark book *Hypothyroidism, the Unsuspected Illness.*[1] During his half-century career as a physician, Barnes observed that *hypothyroidism,* the medical term for an underactive thyroid gland, is far more common than most doctors realize. Furthermore, according to Barnes, standard blood tests used to assess thyroid function are unreliable and often fail to reveal the need for additional thyroid hormone.

SYMPTOMS OF HYPOTHYROIDISM

People with hypothyroidism usually experience one or more of the following: fatigue; depression; trouble concentrating; difficulty getting up in the morning; cold hands and feet; intolerance to cold weather; constipation; thinning hair; fluid retention; dry skin; poor resistance to infection; high cholesterol; premenstrual syndrome; irregular, excessive, or painful menstruation; infertility; fibrocystic breast disease; and ovarian cysts. Although hypothyroidism is certainly not the only cause of these symptoms and problems, it is perhaps the most frequently overlooked cause.

BLOOD TESTS UNRELIABLE

Most doctors today rely on blood tests, such as serum thyroxine (T4), to assess thyroid function. However, the concentration of these hormones in the blood may not necessarily reflect what is going on in the rest of the body. It is well known that tissue resistance to hormones can occur. In other words, even though the concentration of a hormone may be normal in the bloodstream symptoms of a deficiency develop because the body's tissues and organs do not respond properly to the hormonal signal. For example, some diabetics have normal or even elevated levels of insulin. However, they need even more because their cells do not respond adequately to the hormonal message sent by the insulin molecule. This phenomenon, called *insulin resistance,* can be overcome by supplying the body with more insulin. Thyroid hormone resistance has also been described, and may explain why some people with normal blood tests still seem to need more thyroid hormone. The TSH (thyroid stimulating hormone) test, supposedly a more sensitive measure of thyroid function, also appears to miss the diagnosis in many cases.

Barnes discovered that a simple underarm temperature test can be used to predict who will improve with thyroid therapy. If the temperature under your arm in the morning before you get out of bed is 97.4°F or less, and if you have some of the symptoms listed, then you might have hypothyroidism. For women, the temperature should be taken starting the second day of menstruation because considerable temperature fluctuations occur at certain times in the menstrual cycle.

DRAMATIC RESULTS WITH THE BARNES METHOD

Over the past thirteen years, I have used the Barnes approach for more than one thousand patients. Many of these individuals had, in addition to some of the symptoms listed, certain physical signs of hypothyroidism such as dry, coarse skin; puffiness under the eyes and around the ankles; yellowish palms and soles; fluid retention; slowed thinking processes; and delayed Achilles' tendon reflexes. Hundreds of patients have reported that thyroid hormone therapy literally turned their lives around. Problems they had had for years or even decades, problems for which they had consulted numerous physicians without relief, disappeared or improved markedly within days or weeks of beginning thyroid therapy.

A typical case of unsuspected hypothyroidism was H.S., a thirty-seven-year-old woman who came in because of a persistent unexplained cough of more than six months' duration. Additional questioning revealed that her hands and feet were always cold and that for most of her life she had a tendency to fatigue and depression. She also seemed to "catch" any bug that was going around. Despite normal blood tests, thyroid hormone was what worked for her. The cough stopped within days of starting the treatment. When she returned six weeks later she remarked that she never knew anyone could feel as well as she now did. Fatigue and depression, which had for her always been a part of her life, were completely gone. Thyroid hormone allowed her to experience a level of well-being and function that she had never dreamed possible. Years after her initial visit she continues to take thyroid hormone and continues to do well.

Time and again, thyroid therapy has been the answer to years of suffering. As many as 25% of my patients have tried this treatment and, of those, more than half have benefitted. In many cases, thyroid hormone was more effective than any other treatment they had ever tried. Hundreds of my colleagues around the country have seen similar results using the Barnes approach to thyroid therapy. When properly administered, thyroid hormone is remarkably free from side effects. Although a few individuals experience insomnia, rapid pulse, or chest pain which subsides promptly when the treatment is discontinued, not one patient out of the more than one thousand I have treated has had any serious or permanent side effects.

THYROID HORMONE AND OSTEOPOROSIS

So, there it was in 1988, while hundreds of my patients were happily taking thyroid hormone, that a report came along suggesting this treatment could be damaging people's bones. If that were true, then the risk-benefit ratio for thyroid treatment would certainly have to be reevaluated. I imagined having to take some of my patients off of the only treatment that had helped them. Telephone calls started pouring in from worried patients who had heard the report on the news. I wondered how Nolan Ryan would feel if he were not allowed to throw the fastball anymore.

Needless to say, I obtained a copy of the article as fast as possible and studied it carefully. However, I already had a sense that there was something about the report that did not add up. While it had long been known that either hyperthyroidism or administration of excessively large doses of thyroid hormone can cause osteoporosis, no one had ever before suggested that treatment with the usual therapeutic doses of thyroid hormone causes bone loss. Doctors are, in general, a very observant group. They had been prescribing thyroid hormones for more than one hundred years, without ever before associating this treatment with osteoporosis. By contrast, when cortisonelike drugs were first introduced doctors figured out almost immediately that those drugs can ruin your bones. Was it possible that the entire medical profession could have missed a similar effect of thyroid hormone for an entire century, even if the effect was more subtle than that of cortisone?

Because of the importance of this issue, I carefully reviewed all of the relevant studies available. Based on this review, I have concluded that treatment with thyroid hormone in the doses usually prescribed does not cause osteoporosis and does not increase the risk of developing fractures.

The Study

The first study suggesting an association between thyroid hormone and osteoporosis was published in 1988. In that study, bone mineral density was measured in thirty-one women who had been receiving thyroxine (a commonly prescribed thyroid hormone) for an average of 9.6 years. Compared to a control group, bone density at the femur (the site where hip fractures occur) was reduced by anywhere from 10.1% to 12.8%. Bone density at the lumbar spine was similar between the two groups of women. The authors of the study concluded that long-term thyroxine therapy may reduce bone density of the hip.[2]

Problems with the Study

However, there are several reasons to question the conclusions of that study. First, the average dose of thyroxine given to the women was relatively large, 175 mcg per day. Some women were receiving as much as 300 mcg per day, an extremely large amount. Most individuals being treated for an underactive thyroid gland are given between 50 and 150 mcg of thyroxine daily.

Second, and more important, is that the reduction in bone mass observed in thyroxine-treated women may have been due to something other than the treatment. Six of the thirty-one women had previously had Graves' disease, a condition that causes a massive outpouring of thyroid hormones into the bloodstream. This hyperthyroid condition had been treated either by surgically removing the thyroid gland or by destroying it with radioactive iodine. These women were then placed on thyroid hormone, since their thyroid gland was no longer functioning. The problem is that Graves' disease itself can cause osteoporosis. It is therefore inappropriate to blame the bone loss, at least in these six women, on the subsequent treatment.

Another six women in the study had Hashimoto's thyroiditis, an autoimmune disorder in which the immune system attacks the thyroid gland. Hashimoto's disease sometimes causes *hyper*thyroidism until the autoimmune process eventually "burns out" the thyroid gland and causes *hypo*thyroidism. Autoimmune disease is itself often associated with accelerated bone loss. Thus, in the six women with Hashimoto's thyroiditis, the observed reduction in bone mass may have been caused by the disease, not by the subsequent treatment.

The remainder of the thirty-one women studied had been receiving thyroxine to suppress thyroid cancer or other types of nodules (growths) on the thyroid gland. Since women with these conditions do not typically have an underactive thyroid gland in the first place, the extra thyroxine they received to suppress their disease may have been more than their bones could handle. It is also possible that thyroid cancer and thyroid nodules are themselves associated with reduced bone mass. This study does not, therefore, provide any evidence that taking low or moderate doses of thyroid hormones to compensate for an underactive thyroid gland will promote osteoporosis.

Normal Bone Remodeling

In another study, bone mineral density was measured in a group of hypothyroid individuals before and six months after the start of thyroid hormone therapy. Compared to a control group, the rate of bone loss was greater in those receiving thyroid hormone and the rate of bone remodeling was also increased.[3] The authors of the study concluded that treatment with thyroid hormone may result in accelerated bone loss. However, based on what we already know about the relationship between thyroid hormone and bone metabolism, that conclusion is unwarranted.

Confusion surrounding this study is due to the fact that individuals with hypothyroidism tend to have abnormally thick bones.

That is because thyroid hormone is required for normal bone remodeling to take place. As mentioned previously, the purpose of bone remodeling is to replace old bone, damaged by fatigue-fractures from repetitive stress, with newer and stronger bone. Thyroid hormone is one of the triggers for the bone-remodeling cycle, which starts with bone resorption and is followed by new bone formation. If not enough thyroid hormone is present, old bone tends to accumulate—bone that is not necessarily strong or fracture-resistant.

When a hypothyroid individual begins taking thyroid hormone, there will probably be a period of time in which catch-up bone remodeling takes place. Thus, while the bones may be getting slightly thinner (from abnormally dense back to normal), the overall resilience and strength of the bones may actually be improving. An increased rate of bone loss during the first six months of thyroid hormone therapy is therefore no cause for concern. And, there is no evidence that this process continues once the period of catch-up remodeling is over.

NO INCREASED RISK OF BONE LOSS

A study published last year in the *Lancet* demonstrated that thyroid hormone does not, in fact, cause osteoporosis. Bone mineral density was measured at several femoral and vertebral sites in forty-nine patients receiving long-term thyroid hormone (thyroxine) therapy and in a control group matched for age, sex, menopausal status, body mass index, smoking history, and calcium intake. The average duration of thyroxine therapy was 7.9 years and the average dose was 191 mcg/day. The results showed that patients receiving thyroid hormone had no evidence of lower bone mineral density than the controls at any site. Bone mineral density was not correlated with thyroxine dose, duration of therapy, or with tests of thyroid function. These findings, combined with earlier reports that the incidence of fractures is not increased in people taking thyroid hormone, indicate that treatment with thyroid hormone does not cause osteoporosis and does not increase the risk of developing fractures.[4]

CONCLUSION

When all of these studies are considered together, it seems unlikely that treatment with appropriate doses of thyroid hormone will cause osteoporosis. It is certainly important to treat thyroid hormone with respect; take advantage of its powerful benefits when indicated, but always look for the lowest effective dose. If you are taking thyroid hormone, it might be wise to be extra diligent with your osteoporosis-prevention program, just in case. On the other hand, if you have benefitted from thyroid hormone there is no reason at the present time to reduce the dose based on a fear of developing osteoporosis.

NOTES

1. Barnes, B., and Galton, L., 1976. *Hypothyroidism, the unsuspected illness.* New York: Harper & Row.
2. Paul, T. L., et al. 1988. Long-term L-thyroxine therapy is associated with decreased hip bone density in premenopausal women. *JAMA* 259:3137–3141.
3. Coindre, J.-M., et al. 1986. Bone loss in hypothyroidism with hormone replacement. A histomorphometric study. *Arch Intern Med* 146:48–53.
4. Franklin, J. A., et al. 1992. Long-term thyroxine treatment and bone mineral density. *Lancet* 340:9–13.

24

Other Therapies

This book has focused primarily on natural methods of preventing and treating osteoporosis, such as diet, lifestyle, exercise, nutritional supplements, and hormones. It is likely that these interventions alone will be all that is necessary for most women. However, osteoporosis will still develop in some people despite their best efforts. Consequently, drug therapy may be recommended in some cases. Several drugs are currently available that have been shown to have an effect on the process of osteoporosis. The use of these drugs may be considered in cases of severe osteoporosis, where other attempts at treatment have failed.

CALCITONIN

Calcitonin, a hormone composed of thirty-two amino acids, is secreted from the C cells of the thyroid gland. Calcitonin is a potent inhibitor of osteoclasts, the cells that cause bone resorption. In this respect, its action is similar to that of estrogen. Calcitonin levels are lower in women than in men and tend to decrease with advancing age. There is evidence that postmenopausal women with osteoporosis have a lowered reserve of calcitonin, compared to women of similar age without osteoporosis. This deficiency of calcitonin would presumably result in increased bone resorption and accelerated bone loss.

Studies have shown that administering calcitonin increases bone mass in both males and females with osteoporosis. Synthetic calcitonin (Calcimar) has been approved by the Food and Drug Administration for the treatment of postmenopausal osteoporosis. The recommended dosage is 100 MRC units daily by either intramuscular or subcutaneous injection. At a cost of $7.50 per day (or more than $2,700 per year), calcitonin is probably the most expensive treatment for osteoporosis. Side effects include transient facial flushing, nausea with or without vomiting in about 10% of patients treated, and inflammation at the site of injection in about 10% of cases. On rare occasions, calcitonin has caused severe allergic reactions, including anaphylactic shock, and one death due to anaphylaxis has been reported. Despite these side effects, calcitonin is considered a relatively safe drug.

BIPHOSPHONATES

Biphosphonates are synthetic compounds that are chemically similar to pyrophosphate, a compound found naturally in the body composed of phosphorus and carbon. Biphosphonates bind tightly to hydroxyapatite crystals in bone and inhibit bone resorption. In a large randomized trial, 429 women with postmenopausal osteoporosis and vertebral fractures were treated with either etidronate (one of the biphosphonates) or a placebo in a two-year study. Each woman was given either phosphate or a placebo for three days, followed by a placebo or etidronate for fourteen days. All patients were then given 500 mg/day of calcium for seventy-three days. This ninety-day cycle was repeated eight times over a two-year period. The groups receiving etidronate had significant increases in bone mass of the lumbar spine (4.2 to 5.2%) and smaller increases in bone mass at the hip. In addition, there was a significant reduction in the incidence of fractures in those receiving the drug.[1]

Etidronate is sold under the brand name Didronel. It is approved by the Food and Drug Administration for the treatment of a bone disorder, Paget's disease, and to prevent the formation of abnormal calcium deposits following hip replacement surgery. It is not currently approved for the prevention or treatment of osteoporosis. However, regulations concerning prescription drugs state that, if a drug is approved for one purpose physicians may prescribe it for another purpose if, in their judgment, such treatment is warranted. "Off label" uses of prescription drugs are quite common. Side effects of etidronate are rare.

FLUORIDE

Well known for its ability to prevent cavities, fluoride also has an effect on bone metabolism. Fluoride is a potent stimulator of bone formation, and treatment with large doses (such as 30 mg/day) has been shown to increase bone mass in individuals with osteoporosis. However, the new bone growth induced by treatment with large doses of fluoride may not necessarily be high-quality bone, and individuals treated with fluoride sometimes show evidence of abnormalities in their bone tissue. The effect of fluoride on fracture incidence has been studied by a number of different investigators, but the results have been conflicting. A few studies have demonstrated an increased incidence of fractures in people receiving fluoride. Any potential benefit of fluoride treatment must be balanced against reports of serious side effects, including anemia, gastrointestinal symptoms, arthritis, and recurrent vomiting. Given the many other treatments available, administration of large doses of fluoride may not be appropriate for osteoporosis prevention.

WHEN TO USE DRUGS

At the present time, there are no clear guidelines about when to use these treatments. The decision is even more complicated, given the many other natural options described in this book—options that most doctors are still unaware of. As with any treatment, the risks and benefits must be carefully weighed. In my practice, I almost always begin with dietary modifications and nutritional supplements. If severe osteoporosis is already present or if the patient is at high risk for developing it, I might also prescribe hormone therapy. Modern radiologic techniques for measuring bone mass allow us to determine, usually within a year or so, if the treatment is working. If the natural approach is doing what it is supposed to do I will usually continue with it and repeat a bone density study several years later. If bone loss continues, or if the patient experiences additional fractures, I might consider adding drug therapy. Because of its high cost and the need for daily injections, calcitonin is not an acceptable treatment for many patients. Fluoride is not recommended because of its toxicity and because it may increase the risk of some types of fractures. Biphosphonates such as etidronate (Didronel) appear to be the most appropriate medication to use in many circumstances.

PREVENTING FALLS

Although osteoporosis is a prerequisite for many fractures, falling down is often the direct trigger. Colles' fractures of the wrist are nearly always caused when the hands are extended to blunt a fall. Hip fractures in osteoporotic individuals are also frequently a direct result of falling. Taking measures to prevent such falls is therefore very important.

Individuals with osteoporosis should wear comfortable shoes that are easy to walk in. Women should exert caution when walking in heels, particularly when conditions are icy or wet. Those who have an unsteady gait should probably not wear heels at all. If aging or disease results in weakness or frailty, the use of a cane or a walker should be seriously considered. Care should also be taken not to leave objects on the steps or on the floor in places where one might trip over them. Although these recommendations are basically just common sense, they are particularly important for people with osteoporosis.

Beneficial Effect of Potassium

A number of medical conditions increase the likelihood that a person will fall down. One such disorder is called *postural hypotension,* so named because the blood pressure drops excessively when one stands up. Individuals with postural hypotension may become light-headed when they stand up rapidly, causing them to lose their balance and fall down. Postural hypotension is common in the elderly, with 10 to 24% of those over seventy-five years of age exhibiting a fall in systolic blood pressure of 20 mm Hg or more upon standing. Research has shown that individuals with "idiopathic" postural hypotension (that is, where no medical cause of the hypotension was found) have lower concentrations of potassium in their red blood cells than people without this problem.

To determine whether this apparent potassium deficiency plays a causative role, a group of investigators studied the effect of potassium supplements in ten elderly individuals with idiopathic postural hypotension.[2] None of the participants in the study was taking diuretics, a common cause of potassium depletion. Each patient received 60 mmol/day of potassium chloride (equivalent to 2,340 mg/day of potassium) or a placebo, during two separate four-week periods, in a double-blind crossover trial. The average fall in systolic blood pressure upon standing was significantly less (16 mm Hg) during the potassium period than during the placebo period (33 mm Hg).

This study indicates that potassium may be effective in the treatment of idiopathic postural hypotension and might therefore help prevent falls in the elderly. Assuring adequate potassium intake is especially important in people taking certain diuretics, since these drugs are known to deplete potassium. Most fruits and vegetables are good sources of potassium.

Ginkgo Biloba Extract

Some elderly individuals are more likely to sustain a fall because of general unsteadiness or weakness due to their age. Research from Europe has shown that an herbal extract known as Ginkgo biloba extract (GBE), derived from the leaves of the Ginkgo biloba tree, is capable of reversing some of the manifestations of aging, including poor balance.[3] GBE is available in health food stores. It is considered nontoxic and is not known to interact with any prescription drugs. I have also given small doses of DHEA (see Chapter 16) to elderly people suffering from weakness, tremor, and unsteadiness. In some cases, this treatment produces good results.

NOTES

1. Riggs, B. L. 1990. A new option for treating osteoporosis. *N Engl J Med* 323:124–125.
2. Heseltine, D., et al. 1990. Potassium supplementation in the treatment of idiopathic postural hypotension. *Age Ageing* 19:409–414.
3. Vorberg, G. 1985. Ginko biloba extract (GBE): A long-term study of chronic cerebral insufficiency in geriatric patients. *Clin Trials J* 22:149–157.

25

Natural Remedies: The Orphans of the Medical Industry

This book describes some exciting new approaches in the battle against osteoporosis. With each passing year, the evidence grows stronger that we can achieve better results than we are now seeing with the standard calcium/estrogen/exercise approach. It now seems highly likely that a comprehensive program that includes diet, nutritional supplements, avoidance of environmental toxins, and judicious use of natural hormones could prevent a significant proportion of the 1.2 million osteoporotic fractures that occur every year in the United States. Certainly, additional research is needed to confirm and expand upon these initial reports. Hopefully, further studies will also provide us with clearer guidelines about the optimal doses and combinations of the various components of this program. Nevertheless, I believe that currently available evidence is compelling enough to warrant the implementation of new preventive and therapeutic strategies for osteoporosis.

Although it may be many years before we know exactly how beneficial this approach can be, there are many important measures you can take now to fight osteoporosis. Moderating your intake of sugar, caffeine, and alcohol; reducing your exposure to aluminum, lead, cadmium, and tin; and supplementing your diet with the appropriate vitamins and minerals carry little or no risk and do not cost very much. And, even if making these changes turns out not to be as effective against osteoporosis as we had thought, you may realize other benefits, such as more energy and a lower risk of heart disease and cancer. The decision of whether to use the natural hormones DHEA and progesterone is more complicated and should be based on a complete review of your medical history. However, there do appear to be a number of common situations in which the use of these hormones may be advisable, either in addition to or instead of conventional therapy.

CONVENTIONAL MEDICINE RESISTS NEW IDEAS

So, if all of this seems so logical and promising, why is it that so few doctors are providing their patients with the kind of information we are discussing? Why is it that the average doctor is either totally unaware of this work or simply rejects it out of hand as "unproven"? While I can only guess at the reason for the resistance of the medical profession to nutritional and natural therapies, this attitude is certainly not new or unusual. As far back as the eighteenth century, when Sir James Lind discovered the cure for scurvy, his findings were ignored for fifty years. Today, things are often no better.

Several years ago, I received a call from a seventy-seven-year-old woman on a Saturday night, informing me that she was scheduled to have her leg amputated on Monday morning. She wanted to know if there was anything I could do to save her leg. She had had diabetes for a number of years which had greatly impaired the circulation in her legs. After two bypass operations on her right leg had failed and gangrene had appeared in the fourth toe, the doctors decided that the leg must be amputated before bacteria from the toe entered her bloodstream and caused a fatal infection. I had already seen positive results using intravenous magnesium, B-vitamins, and vitamin C to treat gangrene. One such patient who responded to this treatment is presented in Chapter 1. I, therefore, agreed to visit this woman to see if her leg appeared salvageable. After examining her, I felt that immediate amputation was not necessary, and that a trial of intensive nutrient therapy lasting several weeks would be worthwhile.

The patient telephoned her surgeon the next morning and postponed the operation, after informing him that she wished to try nutritional therapy. I immediately received a call from the surgeon, who informed me in no uncertain terms that I was playing with this woman's life and that my treatment obviously could not work, because if it did, everyone would be doing it. I informed the surgeon that I had been able to save the legs of other patients, and cited the patient described in the book's introduction, who had, in fact, been a patient of this same surgeon. He replied that the two cases were different (they were actually quite similar), and reiterated his position that the treatment could not possibly work. He did agree, however, to hospitalize the patient for intravenous antibiotics (I do not do hospital care), so that the nutritional treatment would have a greater chance of succeeding.

On the next to last day of her hospital stay, the surgeon entered her room with a group of residents and medical students and informed the patient that he had scheduled her for amputation the next morning. Somewhat shocked, she replied, "Over my dead body you are," at which time one of the residents, who had obviously been briefed about this "crazy" lady, retorted in a totally condescending and mocking manner, "That's right, you're going to go home and save your leg with vitamins."

The woman did go home and was treated three times a week with intravenous injections of vitamin C, magnesium, and B-complex vitamins. After several weeks, the pain in her leg and toe had diminished substantially. At that time, we decided to have the dead portion of the fourth toe amputated (by another surgeon). But, the portion of the toe above the amputated part appeared pink and perfectly healthy and healed much more rapidly than expected. In addition, there was heavy bleeding from the toe during the procedure, an indication that the circulation had been largely restored by the nutrient injections. The patient continued to receive periodic nutrient injections over the next three years, during which time no new gangrenous lesions appeared.

Although I sent a detailed report of the case to the surgeon, I never heard from him. I also wrote a letter to the education committee at the hospital where both of my patients with gangrenous limbs had been treated. I informed them of my good results and requested permission to speak to their staff about nutrient therapy for circulatory problems. After about two weeks, I was informed that the medical staff at this hospital had "neither the need nor the desire" to hear about nutrient therapy.

As a footnote to this case, the patient was hospitalized a year after the original confrontation with the surgeon. This time, she was being evaluated for stomach pain, not for circulatory problems. However, when the surgeon noticed her name on the hospital admission list, he marched triumphantly to her room and announced that he knew the vitamin treatment would never last. Of course, she informed him that her circulation was fine.

Although not all doctors are known for their good bedside manner, the type of demeaning and abusive behavior described here is particularly common in relation to nutritional medicine or other "alternative" medical practices. In many cases, the anger doctors display is far out of proportion to the situation. For those of us who want to believe that the medical profession is always up on the latest research and always acts in the best interests of the patient, it is disturbing to realize that some doctors are emotionally incapable of hearing the evidence supporting certain treatments.

THE MEDICAL PROFESSION: A DYSFUNCTIONAL FAMILY

It might seem hard to believe that a doctor would consider anything other than the welfare of the patient when formulating his or her recommendations. Most physicians are honorable and dedicated people who would do everything in their power to help their patients. However, being only human, doctors are also motivated by fear and by the natural instinct for self-preservation. And, unfortunately, in the practice of medicine in 1993, there is plenty of fear floating around.

A medical career actually begins as early as the teen years, as the college premed student learns how to scramble for good grades, all the while living in fear of not being accepted into medical school. Once that first hurdle is cleared, many a young adult comes face to face with a system of medical education which is so abusive that it has been compared to a dysfunctional family or even a cult. The life of a medical student is overwhelmed by sleep deprivation, nonnourishing fast food, and an incessant barrage of unverifiable information. On top of all of this, many students are subjected to emotional abuse by residents and professors. Henry K. Silver, M.D., from the University of Colorado School of Medicine, has pointed out the similarities between changes that occur in abused children and those of medical students early in their training. Though they enter medical school eagerly and with enthusiasm, many eventually become cynical, frightened, depressed, and frustrated.

Surveys of medical students reveal that more than 80% experienced being abused at least once during their training. The abuse took many forms. The most common was verbal abuse, in which the student was subjected to inappropriately nasty, rude, or hostile behavior. One-sixth of the students surveyed reported being subjected to actual physical harm, including being slapped, kicked, hit, or having things thrown at them. Nearly one-fifth had experienced a classmate trying to turn a supervisor against them. Eighty-one percent of women reported having been subjected to sexist slurs, most frequently by clinical faculty and house staff. One student felt compelled, because of sexual harassment, to avoid certain physicians. As a result, she was forced to miss some learning opportunities. More than one-third stated that they had seriously considered dropping out of medical school as a result of being mistreated, and many students indicated that the worst episodes of abuse would have an impact on them for the rest of their lives. Furthermore, in addition to the emotional abuse, medical students are also subjected to spiritual abuse, in that they are taught to compare themselves to God and are led to believe they are supposed to know everything.

Under the weight of such pressure and in the interest of

self-preservation, many medical students begin to question their own view of reality and, instead, identify with those who hold power over them. They begin to accept the subtle messages inherent in their standardized medical education, their standardized multiple-choice tests, and their standardized, computerized licensure exams. That message is that there is *one* "acceptable" body of medical knowledge, *one* way to practice medicine, and "standards of care" that must be rigidly adhered to. Since doctors have by this time already been indoctrinated with the notion that they are like God, a nonconformist risks being branded not only an incompetent, but also a heretic. It does not seem to matter that the standards of care were created by fallible human beings whose opinions often, in retrospect, turn out to be quite incorrect.

Tyranny of Conformity

Physicians react to the tyranny of conformity in different ways. To some, the suggestion, for example, that vitamin supplements could help prevent osteoporosis is such a threat to their belief system that they react as if they were being personally attacked. I have encountered many such physicians over the years and long ago I gave up the hope that their minds could be changed. Other doctors acknowledge that there may, indeed, be something to alternative medicine; however, they are unwilling to risk being seen by their colleagues as different.

I once administered chelation therapy to a sixty-five-year-old diabetic who, like the woman just described, had a gangrenous foot which the doctors wanted to amputate. Chelation therapy is a controversial procedure, involving intravenous injections of a drug called EDTA. This drug is approved for the treatment of lead poisoning; however, doctors discovered about forty years ago that it was also a safe and effective treatment for atherosclerosis (hardening of the arteries). More than 500,000 patients have received chelation in the United States. Although this treatment is apparently safer and at least as effective as bypass surgery—and costs 90% less—chelation therapy has never been accepted by conventional medicine. After this patient's leg was saved from amputation by chelation therapy, he asked his cardiologist why he did not utilize this therapy. The cardiologist replied quite frankly, "I make a good living; I'm well respected in the community. Why should I jeopardize it all by doing something so unconventional?"

Some physicians are clearly intrigued by alternative medicine and, on some level, would like to be doing it themselves. However, even they may have great difficulty "taking the plunge" into the realm of nonconformity. I once gave a lecture to a group of local physicians about how thyroid hormone therapy can be useful for a wide range of clinical problems, even in cases where the standard blood tests for thyroid function are normal. (This method of using thyroid hormone is described in more detail in Chapter 23.) Several months later, I received a call from one of the physicians who had attended the lecture. He had a patient who fit the classic picture of hypothyroidism: fatigue, depression, cold extremities, dry skin, constipation, thinning hair, and subnormal body temperature. However, the blood tests for thyroid function were normal. The doctor wanted to refer this patient to me so that I could give her a trial of thyroid hormone. I agreed that such a trial would be worthwhile, but asked the doctor why he did not just prescribe the treatment himself. He replied, with some sadness in his voice, "I'd love to, but my colleagues would rake me over the coals if they found out."

DOUBLE STANDARD

The official excuse used by the medical establishment for rejecting nutritional medicine is that it is "unproven." However, the demand that everything in alternative medicine be "proven" before it can be accepted is truly a double standard. Having studied the medical literature for more than twenty years, I am aware that the scientific support for many aspects of nutritional medicine is as good as, or better than, the evidence in favor of many conventional treatments.

Hundreds of thousands of coronary artery bypass operations are performed every year on heart patients, even though studies have shown time and again that such operations have virtually no

effect on life expectancy. Millions of patients with only mildly elevated cholesterol levels are being advised to take cholesterol-
lowering drugs, despite clear evidence that these drugs do not pro-
long life. Where cancer chemotherapy is concerned, a critical review
published in the *Journal of the American Medical Association*
pointed out that claims for effectiveness are often unwarranted, because they were based on improperly designed studies.[1] Rheuma-
tologists routinely prescribe toxic drugs such as gold, methotrexate,
and hydroxychloroquine (Plaquenil) in the hope of slowing down
the progression of rheumatoid arthritis. However, when pinned
down, arthritis specialists admit that they have no idea whether
these drugs actually influence the long-term outcome of rheumatoid
arthritis. A recent twenty-year study showed that these purported
"disease-modifying" drugs actually do not improve the prognosis of
the disease at all. As a medical student, I was involved in the care
of a patient who was suffering from cerebral edema (swelling of the
brain tissue) resulting from head trauma. As the attending physician
was ordering an intravenous injection of a cortisonelike drug, he
remarked to the students, "We have no scientific evidence that this
helps, which is not to say the treatment is inappropriate."

There are many other examples of accepted medical practices
that cannot in any way be considered proven. Most physicians know
that the practice of medicine is an art, rather than a science. While
scientific data are often helpful, physicians are called upon every day
to make decisions and recommend treatments that cannot be jus-
tified by scientific research. Why, then, do the "authorities" demand
a higher standard where nutritional treatments are concerned. And
why do they often ignore nutritional treatments that *have* fulfilled
the criteria for scientific proof?

Bias against Natural Medicine

It seems that conventional medicine is innately biased against nutritional therapy and other alternative treatments. Physicians who
have spent four years in college, four years in medical school, three
years in a residency program, and two more years in specialty train-

ing want to believe that they are the experts. Someone who has spent thirteen stressful years becoming an expert at administering poisonous chemicals may have a problem with the assertion that there is a simpler and safer approach that any general practitioner can learn. If that claim is true, then why did they waste so many years learning how to juggle toxic drugs? So, in the interest of preserving their status as "expert" and to validate the years they spent in training, many doctors find themselves, perhaps on an unconscious level, rejecting nutritional medicine without ever taking a serious look at it.

The prejudice against nutritional medicine could probably be overcome if it were only a matter of closed-minded doctors looking the other way. However, this bias is far more ingrained, perhaps even institutionalized, throughout many elements of the medical industry. It is seen in medical schools, in medical journal editorial policy, and in standard medical texts. The entire system of medical education has been infiltrated with this bias. Even the economic and political side of the practice of medicine is involved. Insurance companies usually refuse to pay for nutritional therapies. State medical disciplinary boards sometimes censure or take away the license of doctors who practice nutritional medicine. The federal Food and Drug Administration restricts the free flow of information by prohibiting claims to be made about the medicinal value of nutrients and herbs. This multipronged assault makes it incredibly difficult for physicians to practice nutritional medicine, even if they want to.

The antinutrition "consensus" position of the medical establishment often looks more like a conspiracy than a true consensus. The doctors who decide what constitutes the standards of care are usually considered experts by virtue of the fact that they have published a large number of scientific papers. The problem with judging expertise by that criterion is that publishing lots of papers requires obtaining lots of grant money. The sources of funding for nutrition research include the sugar industry, the dairy industry, and various other companies that have a vested interest in a specific point of view. Scientists who are interested in studying the potential adverse effects of sugar and dairy products would certainly not be able to obtain funding from these sources. Conversely, those whose beliefs are in harmony with the corporate goals of the funding sources will be more successful. A former chairman of the department of nutrition at a major university built his career and his "expertise" on research funding from the sugar industry, and paid that industry back by proclaiming there is nothing wrong with sugar.

Medical Journal Bias

The same type of pressure occurs in the publishing of medical journals. For example, the American Society for Clinical Nutrition, publishers of the *American Journal of Clinical Nutrition,* acknowledges at the front of each issue of their journal the "generous support" of certain organizations for "selected educational activities of the Society." The companies that provide this generous support include the Coca-Cola Company, General Foods Corporation, General Mills Foundation, Gerber Products Company, the NutraSweet® Group, the Pillsbury Company, and a host of pharmaceutical companies. Can you imagine these organizations supporting research and education about the damaging effects of all the processed foods they are selling? This type of bias may also extend to the editorial boards that decide which articles will be published and which will be rejected. Many of the individuals on these editorial boards have risen to the top precisely because their philosophy is similar to that of the corporations who provide research funding.

Strong Arm Tactics

This subtle type of bias sometimes becomes more blatant. For example, a former editor of the *Journal of the American Medical Association* (JAMA) alleged that Pfizer, a major pharmaceutical company, had withdrawn $250,000 worth of advertising because an article appearing in *JAMA* had cast one of their drugs in an unfavorable light. Pfizer had also allegedly threatened to cancel an additional $2 million worth of advertising unless *JAMA* published a second article that was more favorable to their drug. Apparently, the editors of *JAMA* acceded to their request.[2]

A large proportion of the medical journals published today could not stay in business without advertising dollars from the pharmaceutical industry. While such strong-arm tactics as those alleged against *JAMA* are probably the exception, there is undoubtedly a more subtle, but more pervasive, type of pressure on editorial boards to keep their sources of funding happy. Since virtually every medical journal advertiser would be displeased by articles emphasizing natural medicine over drugs and surgery, there is little incentive for editorial boards to accept these articles.

I am not implying that those who review manuscripts are corrupt or even conscious of their bias. Nevertheless, doctors and scientists who are interested in nutritional medicine almost invariably complain about how difficult it is to have their work published in "peer-reviewed" medical journals.

Articles on Natural Medicine Rejected

An article recently appeared in the prestigious *New England Journal of Medicine* concerning finasteride (Proscar), a new drug said to be the first effective treatment for benign prostatic hypertrophy (BPH)—enlargement of the prostate. The impending arrival of this drug had been hailed for many months on the financial pages of the *Wall Street Journal,* because Proscar had the potential to be the next billion dollar blockbuster drug for Merck. However, an editorial accompanying the *New England Journal* article, titled "Is the Prostate Pill Finally Here?" stated that the effectiveness of Proscar was not impressive. I had been aware for some time of the use of an extract of saw palmetto berries (botanical name: *Serenoa repens*) to treat BPH. Controlled studies had shown this herbal extract to be safe and effective, and it was considerably less expensive than Proscar. When the report on Proscar appeared in the *New England Journal,* it became clear that Serenoa was also more effective than Proscar. I therefore wrote the following letter to the editor of the *New England Journal:*

October 26, 1992

Editor,
New England Journal of Medicine
10 Shattuck Street
Boston, MA 02115-6094

To the Editor:

The article by Gormley GJ, et al. (1992;327:1185-91) and the accompanying editorial by Lange PH (1992;327:1234-1236) indicate that the effectiveness of finasteride is not impressive.

An attractive alternative treatment for benign prostatic hyperplasia (BPH) is an extract of the plant Serenoa repens (Serenoa; also known as saw palmetto berries), which is available by prescription in Europe and in health food stores in the United States. Like finasteride, Serenoa is an inhibitor of the enzyme 5alpha-reductase. However, Serenoa is not only less expensive, but apparently more effective and safer than finasteride in the treatment of BPH.

In a double-blind trial, 28% of patients receiving Serenoa were rated "greatly improved," compared to none receiving placebo (p < 0.001).[3] Ninety percent of patients had some degree of improvement with Serenoa, compared to only 36% of those given placebo (p < 0.001). The mean urinary flow rate increased relative to placebo by 2.45 ml/second with Serenoa, compared to 1.4 ml/second relative to placebo with finasteride. Furthermore, whereas finasteride failed to decrease residual urine volume, Serenoa reduced mean residual volume from 94.7 to 55.1 ml (p < 0.001).

Impotence, which occurred in approximately 5% of patients taking finasteride, is not a problem with Serenoa. On the contrary, Serenoa is known to herbalists as an aphrodisiac. While the long-term safety of finasteride is unknown, Serenoa has been used safely for decades. It was listed in the *United States Pharmacopoiea* from 1905 to 1926; the *National Formulary* from 1926 to 1950; *The Physicians' Desk Reference* in 1948; *Remington's Practice of Pharmacy,* 10th edition, 1951; and *The*

Homeopathic Pharmacopoiea of the United States, 8th edition, 1979.[4]

Other studies have confirmed the effectiveness of Serenoa in the treatment of BPH.[5,6,7] For those physicians and patients familiar with Serenoa, the question, "Is the prostate pill finally here?" was answered a long time ago.

Sincerely,

Alan R. Gaby, M.D.

After holding onto the letter for nearly three months, and thereby preventing me from submitting it to another journal, the editors sent a rejection notice, stating that they did not have enough space to print the letter in their journal. How ironic that they had found it appropriate to publish a six-page article and an editorial about a drug that does not work very well, but could not allocate one-quarter of one page to an herbal extract that works better, costs a lot less, and is safer. Because of this editorial bias, the tens of thousands of physicians who read the *New England Journal* were deprived of the opportunity to learn about a better treatment for their patients.

FDA Prohibits Free Flow of Information

This censoring of information about natural alternatives is not limited to medical journals. The Food and Drug Administration (FDA) has a policy that makes it extremely difficult for anyone to learn about the health benefits of natural substances. According to the FDA's interpretation of the law, any substance for which a health claim is made becomes a drug, subject to the same strict rules and regulations as prescription pharmaceuticals. For a substance to be approved by the FDA for a certain medical condition it must pass a rigorous series of tests that can cost more than $50 million to perform. Because natural products do not enjoy patent protection, no one is willing to invest the money to put them through the FDA approval process.

Consequently, very few vitamins, minerals, plant extracts, or other natural compounds have ever been approved by the FDA. Although most of these products can be sold in health food stores and pharmacies, it is illegal for the manufacturer to tell you what conditions they may be helpful for. An "unapproved" health claim immediately causes the product to be classified as a "misbranded drug," subject to seizure by the FDA. Even the presence of books, tapes, scientific papers, or other educational material in the same store has been interpreted as a "claim," if that material contains information pertaining to the medicinal value of products sold in the store.

Over the years, the FDA has enforced this policy with a vengeance. Safe and effective natural remedies, such as Coenzyme Q_{10} and evening primrose oil, have been seized from health food stores or distributors because the FDA did not approve of the statements being made about them. Those seizures were rather peculiar, in view of the massive body of scientific research attesting to the value of each of these substances. Coenzyme Q_{10} has been shown to be of great value in the treatment of congestive heart failure, cardiomyopathy (a disease of the heart muscle), high blood pressure, periodontal disease, and even immune system-related conditions such as AIDS. Evening primrose oil has shown promise in the treatment of eczema, high blood pressure, arthritis, and possibly even multiple sclerosis. The reports on which these "claims" were made are available in any medical school library. Nevertheless, the FDA decided to seize these products because someone was disseminating this information to the public.

The FDA has also engaged in a biased and unfair policy against the herbal extract Serenoa, discussed earlier, as a treatment for prostatic enlargement. Even though this product has been used in this country for nearly one hundred years, the FDA arbitrarily chose to classify it as a new drug. Consequently, no one was allowed to say it was good for the prostate, even though all the old herbal books were already saying that. In late 1992, the FDA prohibited Biotherapeutics, Ltd., a major distributor of Serenoa, from selling their product. The FDA objected to the name of the product, Prostaril, which sounded too much like "prostate" and, therefore, constituted a claim for the product.

FDA RAIDS MEDICAL CLINIC

The FDA has, at times, engaged in even more horrifying tactics. On May 6, 1992, FDA agents, backed up by local police, pulled a Gestapo-like armed raid on the Tahoma Medical Clinic in Kent, Washington. Breaking down the front door and entering wearing flak jackets, they terrified the secretaries and medical staff with drawn guns. For the next fourteen hours, the FDA agents proceeded to seize various vitamins, minerals, patient charts, diagnostic equipment, and educational material. The Tahoma Clinic, operated by Jonathan V. Wright, M.D., has provided state-of-the-art nutritional treatment to thousands of patients. Dr. Wright is considered one of the world's experts in nutritional biochemistry.

Dr. Wright had originally incurred the wrath of the FDA by refusing to adhere to their ban on tryptophan, an essential amino acid shown to be effective in the treatment of depression and insomnia. In 1989, a manufacturing error by a Japanese company resulted in the distribution of a contaminated batch of tryptophan, which caused hundreds of toxic reactions and several dozen deaths. Before these reactions were traced to a contaminant, the FDA banned the sale of tryptophan tablets. However, when the cause of the problem was determined, numerous physicians and many individuals who had benefitted from tryptophan felt that it should be legalized again. After all, prior to the contamination episode, tryptophan had been used for more than twenty-five years, without any hint of serious side effects. Had not the FDA reapproved Tylenol after the cyanide contamination incident? However, much to the delight of the makers of antidepressants and sleeping pills, the FDA refused to let tryptophan back on the market.

Dr. Wright questioned the authority of the FDA to continue its ban on uncontaminated tryptophan. He, therefore, obtained a batch of tryptophan, had it certified by the Mayo Clinic as uncontaminated, and dispensed it to patients in his clinic who needed it. Many of these patients were seriously depressed and had either failed to respond to antidepressant medication or could not tolerate it. Tryptophan, on the other hand, had been effective for them and free of side effects. When the FDA learned that Wright was dispensing tryptophan they came to his office and seized his entire supply. Wright subsequently filed a lawsuit against the FDA, asking for the return of his property and that the FDA cease any further harassment of his clinic.

Shortly thereafter, in August of 1991, FDA agents began rummaging through the dumpster outside of the Tahoma Clinic, looking for evidence to use against Dr. Wright and his clinic. According to an affidavit filed by the FDA to obtain a search warrant (not a guns-drawn commando raid), these late-night dumpster investigations turned up, among other things, injectable B-vitamins from Germany which, according to the FDA, were misbranded drugs. Wright was using German injectable vitamins in his clinic because many of his patients were allergic to the preservatives found in American injectable vitamins. Germany is apparently the only place in the world where high quality preservative-free injectable B-vitamins can be obtained. However, according to the FDA, the product was misbranded because the package insert was not in English. The FDA used this and other "evidence" as an excuse for trashing the Tahoma Clinic in a raid that has since come to be known as "The Great B-Vitamin Bust."

Harassment by State Medical Boards

Harassment by regulatory authorities is not limited to the FDA. A number of state medical disciplinary boards have censured or revoked the license of doctors whose only crime was to emphasize natural remedies over drugs and surgery. These types of actions against qualified practitioners have been going on for years, and a number of cases are pending as this book goes to press.

So it is that the medical establishment, supported by the regulatory authorities, set it up so that doctors risk a great deal if they do not follow the rules. That type of mindset makes it very difficult for a doctor to try treatments outside of the mainstream. With respect to hormones such as estriol and DHEA the resistance is even greater because these substances are not officially approved by the FDA. While it is legal for a physician to prescribe these natural compounds many doctors are reluctant to do so without the official "blessing" of the FDA.

WHO BENEFITS?

Who benefits from this monopoly situation in which many safe, effective, and inexpensive treatments are suppressed? Certainly not the public. The pharmaceutical industry benefits because it is able to enjoy a greater monopoly for its patented medications. The so-called authorities in the medical establishment benefit because their pronouncements carry greater weight. And the medical profession in general also profits because the public is kept in the dark about effective treatments that anyone can buy in a health food store without a prescription. I do not think there is a conscious conspiracy between these arms of the medical industry to suppress natural medicine. However, those who profit from the current situation are usually able to find a way to rationalize what they are doing.

In 1985, the Pharmaceutical Advertising Council teamed up with the FDA to solicit funds from the pharmaceutical industry for the purpose of combatting medical quackery. According to their definition, quackery includes the therapeutic use of vitamins. A large number of drug companies donated to that cause. It is unlikely that those involved in that fund drive were purposely trying to harm the public. They may have been genuinely interested in stopping the exaggerated claims that sometimes emanate from the health food industry. Nevertheless, campaigns like that make it more difficult for the truth to be told about those aspects of nutritional medicine that have been well documented and that are clearly effective.

ORPHANS OF THE MEDICAL INDUSTRY

Thus, the medicinal products found in nature remain the orphans of the medical industry. Fortunately, however, things are beginning to change. The FDA raid on the Tahoma Clinic and several earlier raids on nutritional supplement manufacturers have created public outrage and have led to the formation of a number of political action groups. The Nutritional Health Alliance (1-800-226-4NHA) and the American Preventive Medical Association (206-926-0551) are heavily involved in promoting public awareness of the problems and are supporting much needed changes in the law. Partly because of the work of these groups, Congress is considering legislation that will increase the freedom of the public to obtain the type of health care they desire and of doctors to deliver the kind of health care they believe is in the best interests of their patients. Much more work needs to be done. However, it is hoped that one day soon, information such as that presented in this book can be judged solely on its own merits, without the damaging influence of fear.

NOTES

1. Oye, R. K., and M. F. Shapiro. 1984. Reporting results from chemotherapy trials. Does response make a difference in patient survival? *JAMA* 252:2722–2725.
2. Anonymous. 1984. Journal said to bow to drug advertiser. *Baltimore Sun,* 15 January.
3. Champault, G., J. C. Patel, and A. M. Bonnard. 1984. A double-blind trial of an extract of the plant Serenoa repens in benign prostatic hyperplasia. *Br J Clin Pharmacol* 18:461–462.
4. *Federal Register.* 1990. 42,434–42,442.
5. Cirillo-Marucco, E., et al. 1983. Extract of Serenoa repens (Permixon) in the early treatment of prostatic hypertrophy. *Urologia* 50:1269–1277.
6. Tripodi, V., et al. 1983. Treatment of prostatic hypertrophy with Serenoa repens extract. *Med Praxis* 4:41–46.
7. Emili, E., M. Lo Cigno, and U. Petrone. 1983. Clinical trial of a new drug for treating hypertrophy of the prostate (Permixon). *Urologia* 50:1042–1048.

26

Natural Remedies for
Women's Health Problems

As many as 75% of all visits to doctors are by women. This statistic has been interpreted to mean that women are either (1) more delicate and more susceptible to illness than men, (2) bigger complainers, or (3) more in tune with their bodies than the opposite sex. Whatever the reason for the greater number of doctor's visits, it has been argued that the treatment of women by doctors leaves much to be desired. For example, in one study, when a group of men and women came to the doctor with identical complaints, significantly more tests were ordered on the men than on the women. This study suggests that many doctors take women's complaints less seriously than they do men's. Another problem is that most of the research pertaining to certain medical conditions (particularly heart disease) has been done exclusively on men. As a result, the recommended treatment for these diseases may not necessarily be applicable to women, whose hormonal system and metabolism differ substantially from that of men.

With increasing public awareness of women's health issues and with the increase in the number of female physicians, the medical care offered to women is beginning to improve. However, we still have a long way to go. As with medicine in general, natural and holistic treatments for women have been slow to find their way into the mainstream. Nevertheless, many of the health conditions encountered by women can be controlled by nontoxic interventions, such as dietary modification and the use of nutritional supplements and other natural substances. Because this approach is safer and frequently more effective than what conventional doctors have to offer, natural medicine should be taken more seriously.

Although this is a book about osteoporosis, I thought it would be worthwhile to discuss other common women's health problems. The information that follows is a compilation of research published over the past fifty years, combined with the personal experience of the author.

GENERAL PRINCIPLES

1. **Cleaning up the diet**   Many women's bodies are intolerant to refined sugar, caffeine, and alcohol, the three major toxins in the American diet. Symptoms these substances may cause include fatigue, depression, anxiety, headaches, insomnia, joint pains, premenstrual syndrome, fibrocystic breasts, and gastrointestinal symptoms. Because sugar, caffeine, and alcohol are all addictive substances, it may be difficult to eliminate them from the diet. I inform my patients that the period of addiction withdrawal (causing primarily irritability and headaches) is usually only 3 to 5 days, after which chronic symptoms should start to improve. Many people find that taking extra vitamin C, magnesium, chromium, vitamin B-complex, and other supplements helps them make it through the period of withdrawal with fewer symptoms. Thereafter, chronic complaints begin to improve usually within 5 to 14 days after the dietary changes have been made.

2. **Food allergies**   Chronic conditions, such as asthma, recurrent infections, nasal congestion, arthritis, frequent urina-

tion, irritable bowel syndrome, migraines, fatigue, and depression, may be caused entirely or in part by allergies to commonly consumed foods. Food allergies are typically hidden or masked, in that the allergic individual is not aware of a cause–effect relationship between eating certain foods and specific symptoms. However, during a three-week elimination diet (no sugar, coffee, tea, alcohol, corn, eggs, wheat, dairy products, citrus, or food additives), chronic symptoms often disappear and the food allergies become "unmasked." Challenges with individual foods may then produce rapid and exaggerated reactions. By avoiding the symptom-provoking foods, allergic individuals can control many chronic symptoms. Food allergies are discussed in more detail in Chapter 17 and Appendix B.

3. **Hypothyroidism**   Some doctors believe that hypothyroidism (underactive thyroid gland) is very common and that this condition is usually misdiagnosed. According to Broda Barnes, M.D., as many as 40% of all Americans are hypothyroid, compared to an estimated 3% reported in most standard textbooks. In my experience, using the Barnes method of diagnosis, at least 15% of the women who come to my office benefit from taking thyroid hormone. Symptoms of an underactive thyroid may include fatigue, depression, fluid retention, constipation, cold extremities, dry skin, confusion, trouble concentrating, menstrual irregularities, and infertility. The Barnes method of diagnosing hypothyroidism is described in Chapter 23.

Although blood tests for thyroid function are usually normal, certain clues may be found on a careful physical examination. These include delayed Achilles tendon reflexes, dry and flaky skin, and puffiness under the eyes and around the ankles. The skin may also be yellowish, resulting from inefficient conversion of beta-carotene to vitamin A. The presence of a subnormal body temperature provides an additional clue to possible hypothyroidism. If the situation warrants, a trial of thyroid hormone may be initiated. In many cases, thyroid hormone is the only treatment that helps the symptoms.

A large proportion of the symptoms that women have can be effectively controlled by these simple modalities: avoiding sugar, caffeine, and alcohol; eliminating allergenic foods from the diet; and judiciously using low dosages of thyroid hormone. In addition, many nonspecific complaints also improve with a broad-spectrum multiple-vitamin and mineral supplement.

TREATMENT OF SPECIFIC CONDITIONS

Leg Cramps During Pregnancy

Leg cramps that occur during pregnancy may improve with supplements of calcium[1] and magnesium. However, drinking extra milk does not help leg cramps, as there is too much phosphorus relative to calcium in milk. In fact, in one study, leg cramps occurring during pregnancy actually became more severe when women increased their milk intake, but were eliminated by reducing milk consumption.[2]

Toxemia During Pregnancy

Toxemia during pregnancy is a condition in which fluid retention, high blood pressure, and spillage of protein into the urine develops late in pregnancy. If toxemia becomes severe, it can cause seizures and possible harm to both the mother and the infant. Toxemia during pregnancy may be prevented by consuming a diet high in protein and by taking supplements containing vitamin B6. In a study published in1956, pregnant women at term had laboratory evidence of vitamin B6 deficiency. This deficiency was more marked in women with toxemia than in those with normal pregnancies. To determine whether vitamin B6 deficiency played a role in toxemia, 820 women were given a daily multivitamin containing either 10 mg of vitamin B6 or no vitamin B6. There was a 61% reduction in the incidence of toxemia in the group given vitamin B6, compared to the control group (1.7% vs. 4.4%).[3] Other studies have shown that extra calcium and magnesium may help prevent toxemia of pregnancy. The conventional treatment of toxemia is to give large doses of magnesium intravenously when the condition becomes severe. However, by using these preventive measures, this heroic "rescue" with intravenous magnesium would be needed much less often.

Nausea and Vomiting During Pregnancy

According to a recent report and many studies from the 1950s, vitamin B6 supplements reduce the severity of nausea and vomiting caused by pregnancy. The dose used in most studies was 50 mg/day. Larger doses should not be used during pregnancy without medical supervision. When vitamin B6 does not work, a combination of vitamin K and vitamin C may be effective. In a study published in 1952, seventy women with nausea and vomiting during pregnancy received 25 mg of vitamin C and 5 mg of a synthetic form of vitamin K (menadione bisulfite) daily for an average of thirty days. Sixty-four women (91%) reported complete relief of symptoms within seventy-two hours and an additional three patients were relieved of vomiting, but continued to have nausea. Vitamin C alone produced little or no benefit and vitamin K alone was helpful in only 50% of the cases. The combination of these vitamins was considerably more effective than either alone.[4] Although this study was published in the *American Journal of Obstetrics and Gynecology,* very few obstetricians today know about it.

Preventing Neural Tube Defects

Spina bifida, a defect in the closure of the fetal neural tube, occurs in about 0.2% of live births. It has now been clearly shown that folic acid supplementation prior to and during the first thirty days of pregnancy will reduce the incidence of neural tube defects by about 80%. Since the neural tube closes around the second week of gestation (before most women even know they are pregnant), folic acid supplements should be started as soon as a pregnancy is planned. Public health authorities are now recommending that all women of childbearing age ingest 0.4 mg/day of folic acid (see Chapter 6 for additional discussion).

Postpartum Depression

Many women experience moderate or severe depression following the birth of a child. Although this condition is complex and has both physical and psychological causes, a high proportion of women with postpartum depression respond rapidly either to thyroid hormone or to intramuscular injections of vitamin B12 and folic acid.

Fibrocystic Breast Disease

Fibrocystic breast disease (also known as cystic mastitis or mammary dysplasia) is so common that some physicians do not think it should be called a disease. Nevertheless, a substantial proportion of American women have cysts in their breasts. Some cysts are painful, whereas others are not. Although it has been suggested that fibrocystic breast disease increases the risk of breast cancer, there is no proof that that is true.

Studies have shown that elimination of caffeine from the diet is frequently of great benefit to women who have cystic breasts. In most cases, merely cutting down on the caffeine does not help very much; complete avoidance is necessary to achieve good results. Common sources of caffeine include coffee, tea, cola beverages, and certain pain medications. In addition, chocolate contains a caffeine-like compound, which may have similar adverse effects on breast tissue. Supplementation with vitamin E and thiamine (vitamin B1) are also helpful in some cases. Thyroid hormone and evening primrose oil have also been used with some success.

Perhaps the most effective nutritional remedy is a solution containing elemental iodine. In one study, 143 women with fibrocystic breasts received 3 to 6 mg/day of iodine by mouth. Of this group, 72% had complete resolution of the problem and an additional 27.5% had marked improvement within three months. At the present time, the form of iodine used in this study is not commercially available. However, some innovative physicians are asking their pharmacists to compound a similar formula and the results appear to be good. Other forms of iodine are sold in the drug store, but not all are suitable for human consumption. Any attempt at iodine therapy should therefore be undertaken only under medical supervision.

Premenstrual Syndrome

It has been estimated that as many as 70 to 90% of women of childbearing age have premenstrual syndrome (PMS), which is defined as recurrent symptoms occurring prior to menstruation. The symptoms can range from mild to severe and include anxiety, depression, intestinal bloating, headaches, acne flareups, weight gain, fluid retention, swollen and painful breasts, and cravings for sweets and salt. These symptoms generally occur the same time each month and can last anywhere from one day to two weeks.

Many women with PMS find that eliminating sugar, caffeine, and alcohol from their diet results in an improvement in symptoms. Some women also seem to be sensitive to dairy products and do better when they avoid them. Research has shown that aerobic exercise also reduces the severity of PMS. In one study, women who ran 1.5 miles daily, five days a week had significant improvements in premenstrual symptoms. Nutritional supplements have also been shown to be beneficial. The most important nutrients are vitamin B6, magnesium, vitamin E, and essential fatty acids. According to one study, a fairly large proportion of women with PMS have subtle hypothyroidism, and treatment with thyroid hormone results in symptom relief. In my experience, most women have a satisfactory response to diet, nutritional supplements, exercise and, when appropriate, thyroid hormone.

In the occasional woman who does not improve with this approach natural progesterone is often helpful. Although controlled studies have failed to show a beneficial effect of progesterone for

PMS, proponents of this treatment argue that these studies were not done properly. I have treated about thirty patients with PMS using natural progesterone and the vast majority felt it was helpful. According to Christiane Northrup, M.D., an expert in women's health care, progesterone is most helpful for women whose PMS symptoms begin suddenly, almost as if a light has been turned off.

Abnormal Menstruation

Abnormal menstruation can take many forms. Some women have a complete absence of menstrual periods (amenorrhea), whereas others menstruate less frequently than normal (oligomenorrhea). For some women, menstruation is excessively heavy (menorrhagia); for others, spotting occurs between periods (metrorrhagia). Excessive menstrual cramping is known as dysmenorrhea. Anyone with menstrual abnormalities should have a thorough gynecologic checkup. However, gynecologists typically overlook some simple, safe, and effective natural remedies for menstrual dysfunction. If the doctor is unable to find a cause for any of the menstrual disorders described here, there is a good chance they may be caused by subtle hypothyroidism. Doctors who use the Barnes method of diagnosing hypothyroidism (see Chapter 23), frequently find that these problems disappear with thyroid hormone therapy.[5]

Vitamin A has also been used successfully to treat menorrhagia. In a study from Australia, serum vitamin A levels were found to be significantly lower in seventy-one women with menorrhagia than in healthy controls. Forty of the women with menorrhagia were given 50,000 units of vitamin A daily for fifteen days. Among these women, menstruation returned to normal in 57.5% and improved substantially in an additional 35%. Thus, 92.5% of the women receiving vitamin A had either complete relief or significant improvement in their excessive menstrual bleeding.[6] Vitamin A at a dosage of 50,000 units/day for fifteen days is nontoxic. However, prolonged administration of vitamin A at this dosage could cause toxicity and should be medically supervised.

Another possible cause of excessive menstrual bleeding is iron deficiency.[7] Iron has a number of important functions in the body in addition to its blood-building role. Iron is necessary for normal muscle contraction, including the muscles of the uterus. When shedding of the uterine lining results in menstrual bleeding the uterine muscles clamp down on the blood vessels, thereby minimizing the amount of blood lost. In the face of iron deficiency, uterine muscle contraction may be impaired and excessive bleeding may occur. Ironically, heavy bleeding is an important cause of iron deficiency, which may, in turn, make the bleeding even worse. In mild cases, oral iron supplements may break this vicious cycle. However, when severe iron deficiency accompanies excessive menstrual blood loss a series of intramuscular iron injections may be necessary.

Women who suffer from bleeding between periods (metrorrhagia) may respond to supplementation with vitamin C combined with bioflavonoids (a group of compounds found in fruits, vegetables, and some other plants).[8] These nutrients improve the integrity of the capillaries, making it more difficult for blood to leak through them.

Women with abnormal menstrual bleeding should always consult a doctor before trying any of these remedies. Serious causes of abnormal bleeding (such as cancer) must be ruled out.

Cervical Dysplasia (Abnormal Pap Smears)

Death from cervical cancer is almost entirely preventable if cervical dysplasia (precancerous changes of the cervix) are detected early by routine Pap smears. As discussed in Chapter 6, treatment with large doses of folic acid may prevent or reverse cervical dysplasia. Preliminary studies have suggested that high intakes of vitamin A[9] and vitamin C[10] may also be helpful. It is important to remember that adequate follow-up of abnormal Pap smears is essential, even if you are taking the vitamins and minerals listed here.

Endometriosis

Endometriosis is a disorder in which uterine tissue grows in areas outside of the uterus. The cause of this painful condition is not known, although it is believed to be related to excess levels of estrogen in the body. Because the liver is responsible for breaking down estrogen, it has been suggested that a weakness in the liver may be one of the causes of endometriosis. At a recent medical conference, a naturopathic physician reported the cases of fifteen women with endometriosis who were treated with an herbal preparation known to stimulate liver function. The formula contained dandelion root, beet leaves, Cascara sagrada, Parsley leaf powder, and Uva ursi. After several months, 12 of the 15 women were free of the pain of endometriosis.

Yeast Infections

Some women suffer from recurrent or persistent vaginal yeast infections. Frequent yeast infections may result from diabetes or from some other medical conditions; however, most of the time no specific cause is found. Experience has shown that eliminating refined carbohydrates from the diet (including all sweets and fruit juices) may help prevent recurrences of yeast infections. Food allergies may cause inflammation of the vaginal mucous membranes, rendering them more susceptible to yeast infections. Women who have recurrent yeast infections often find that, by avoiding the foods to which they are allergic, they are no longer plagued by this persistent problem. In some cases, dietary changes alone are not sufficient and oral antiyeast medications, such as nystatin, ketoconazole (Nizoral), or fluconazole (Diflucan), are necessary.

There is currently much debate about the existence of the *candida-related complex* (CRC). The theory among some physicians is that the intestinal tract can be a major site for yeast growth; that the yeast germ *Candida albicans* produces toxins that are absorbed into the body; and that these toxins can cause a wide range of symptoms including fatigue, depression, spaciness, bloating, diarrhea, headaches, and muscle aches. More serious diseases such as multiple sclerosis and lupus have also been attributed to yeast in some cases. My own clinical experience confirms that CRC is a true clinical entity and that it can cause any of these symptoms. However,

I have also seen many patients who have erroneously attributed their symptoms to candida. Yeast infections are not the cause of everything and blaming everything on yeast sometimes impedes the process of getting well.

The diagnosis of CRC may be difficult because lab tests are unreliable. Effective treatments include dietary modifications and the use of antiyeast medications. Taking Lactobacillus acidophilus (the bacteria found naturally in yogurt) may help repopulate the intestines with friendly bacteria, making it more difficult for candida to thrive. Eating yogurt has also been shown to prevent recurrent vaginal yeast infections. Chronic yeast problems are often triggered by taking antibiotics, birth control pills, or corticosteroids (cortisonelike drugs).

Menopausal Symptoms

Hot flashes and depression are common symptoms associated with menopause. Estrogen replacement therapy (discussed in Chapter 14) usually relieves these symptoms. But, because of its potential side effects, some women wish to avoid using estrogen. Certain natural alternatives to estrogen exist, but none are universally effective. Soybeans contain certain natural substances, phytoestrogens, that have estrogen-like activity; they may account for the rarity of menopausal symptoms in countries such as Japan, where large amounts of soy products are consumed. Calcium, magnesium, folic acid, vitamin E, and bioflavonoids, have also been recommended to prevent or treat menopausal symptoms. Ginseng also has estrogenlike activity and some women find it helpful for alleviating menopausal symptoms. However, ginseng should be treated with respect; an overdose can cause high blood pressure, anxiety, and other side effects.

Breast Cancer

The most serious health concern women in America face today is breast cancer. According to current statistics, breast cancer will develop in 1 of every 9 women in this country. Numerous studies have demonstrated a relationship between nutrition and breast cancer. It is now well documented that women who consume a high-fat diet are at increased risk. Research from the University of Maryland suggests that a specific type of fat, known as trans-fatty acids, is the most significant contributor to breast cancer risk. Foods high in trans-fatty acids include margarine and baked goods that contain partially hydrogenated vegetable oil. Other research suggests that margarine is no safer for the heart than butter, even though margarine is free of cholesterol. I therefore advise my patients to use butter in moderation and to avoid margarine completely.

Another recent study demonstrated that the content of PCBs (polychlorinated biphenyls) and other potentially carcinogenic chemicals in the tissues of women with breast cancer is 50% to 60% higher than in healthy women.[11] These chemicals concentrate at the top of the food chain in animal foods such as meat, eggs, and milk, with the highest concentrations found in the fatty portions of the foods. It is therefore possible that the association between dietary fat intake and breast cancer is due to the presence of carcinogenic chemicals in animal fat. If that is the case, then eating a more vegetarian diet would reduce the risk of developing breast cancer. Excess alcohol consumption has also been associated with an increased risk of breast cancer. Although caffeine intake is one cause of fibrocystic breasts, a relationship between caffeine and breast cancer has not been proven.

A number of individual nutrients have been reported either in animal experiments or in human epidemiologic studies to reduce the risk of breast cancer. These include vitamin C, vitamin E, selenium, and iodine. Other nutrients that may help prevent cancer in general are beta-carotene, zinc, and magnesium. Although supplementing the diet is no guarantee against cancer, I often recommend moderate doses of these nutrients as an "insurance policy."

NOTES

1. Hammar, M., L. Larsson, and L. Tegler. 1981. Calcium treatment of leg cramps in pregnancy. *Acta Obstet Gynecol Scand* 60:345–347.

2. Page, E. W., and E. P. Page. 1953. Leg cramps in pregnancy: Etiology and treatment. *Obstet Gynecol* 1:94–100.

3. Wachstein, M., and L. W. Graffeo. 1956. Influence of vitamin B6 on the incidence of preeclampsia. *Obstet Gynecol* 8:177–180.

4. Merkel, R. L. 1952. The use of menadione bisulfite and ascorbic acid in the treatment of nausea and vomiting of pregnancy: A preliminary report. *Am J Obstet Gynecol* 64:416–418.

5. Stoffer, S. S. 1982. Menstrual disorders and thyroid insufficiency: Intriguing cases suggesting an association. *Postgrad Med* 72(2):75–82.

6. Lithgow, D. M., and W. M. Politzer. 1977. Vitamin A in the treatment of menorrhagia. *S Afr Med J* 51:191–193.

7. Taymor, M. L., S. H. Sturgis, and C. Yahia. 1964. The etiological role of chronic iron deficiency in production of menorrhagia. *JAMA* 187:323–327.

8. Cohen, J. D., and H. W. Rubin. 1960. Functional metrorrhagia: Treatment with bioflavonoids and vitamin C. *Curr Ther Res* 2:539–542.

9. Wylie-Rosett, J. A., et al. 1984. Influence of vitamin A on cervical dysplasia and carcinoma in situ. *Nutr Cancer* 6(1):49–57.

10. Anonymous. 1983. Vitamin C may help prevent cervical dysplasia. *Family Pract News*, 1–14 March, 26.

11. Falck, F., Jr., et al. 1992. Pesticides and polychlorinated biphenyl residues in human breast lipids and their relation to breast cancer. *Arch Environ Health* 47:143–145.

27

Summary and Recommendations

This book has presented information on how to prevent and reverse osteoporosis. Much of what has been discussed is based on exciting new research. Some of the information, on the other hand, is relatively old, though important, data overlooked or ignored by the so-called authorities in the field of osteoporosis. Standard review articles and textbooks on osteoporosis have focused almost exclusively on the importance of calcium, vitamin D, estrogen, exercise, and drugs such as calcitonin, biphosphonates, and fluoride. Most of these sources also recognize the importance of limiting the use of alcohol and tobacco.

There is no question that the conventional approach to osteoporosis prevention has value. However, the limitations of this viewpoint are inherent in the "conventional wisdom" that osteoporosis cannot be reversed or even prevented, but, rather, can only be delayed. The evidence I have discussed in this book indicates that we can do much better than that. And the fact that 1.2 million osteoporotic fractures still occur every year in this country highlights the need for implementing new ideas. The results of published research strongly suggest that a comprehensive program that includes diet, lifestyle, nutritional supplements, a more complete and more physiologic (natural) approach to hormone replacement therapy, and avoidance of certain environmental toxins can produce results that the average doctor does not realize are possible. Additional research is needed, both to facilitate acceptance of these new ideas by the medical establishment, and to help us fine-tune our recommendations. However, on the basis of what is already known, a number of recommendations can be made.

DIETARY RECOMMENDATIONS

An osteoporosis-prevention diet should restrict refined sugar, caffeine, and alcohol. Protein intake should be moderate, in contrast to some American diets which contain excessive amounts of protein. Salt should also be used in moderation, since there is evidence that some individuals lose calcium from their body if they ingest too much salt. Whole grains should be used instead of refined grains because refining of grains results in substantial losses of many of the vitamins and minerals needed to maintain healthy bones. Heavily processed foods should also be avoided, since processing may destroy important nutrients. Cola beverages, which contain excessive amounts of phosphorus (not to mention too much sugar and caffeine in most cases) should also be avoided, since too much phosphorus may adversely affect calcium metabolism.

NUTRITIONAL SUPPLEMENTS

Even if your diet emphasizes wholesome, nutrient-rich foods, supplementing with vitamins and minerals may be worthwhile. It is sometimes forgotten that bone is living tissue, with a wide range of nutritional needs. Failure to meet any one of a number of different nutritional requirements could promote osteoporosis. It is difficult to obtain the Recommended Dietary Allowance (RDA) for certain nutrients from diet alone. Furthermore, because of genetic factors, combined with the effects of stress and environmental pollution, some individuals may need more than the RDA for particular nutrients to achieve optimal bone health. Although it is not possible to determine exactly how much of each nutrient a person needs (the requirement certainly varies from person to person), we do have enough information to make interim recommendations. For individuals wishing to take supplements to reduce their risk of osteoporosis, the range of suggested daily dosages follows:

Minerals

Calcium	400–1,200 mg
Magnesium	200–600 mg
Zinc	10–30 mg
Copper	1–2 mg
Manganese	5–20 mg
Boron	1–3 mg
Silicon	1–2 mg
Strontium	0.5–3 mg

Vitamins

Vitamin B6	5–50 mg
Folic acid	0.4–5 mg
Vitamin C	100–1,000 mg
Vitamin D	100–400 units
Vitamin K	100–500 mcg

Remember that some dosages are listed in milligrams (mg), whereas others are listed in micrograms (mcg; 1 mg = 1,000 mcg).

These levels of nutrients are safe for the average healthy individual and are likely to correct nearly all deficiencies, as well as meet most requirements that are higher than normal. A number of multiple-vitamin and mineral products on the market provide most or all of the nutrients listed in appropriate amounts. Several precautions are in order, however, if you are taking these supplements. First, individuals who are taking the blood-thinning drugs coumadin or warfarin should not take vitamin K, as it interferes with the anticoagulant effect of the drugs. Vitamin K does not, on the other hand, interfere with heparin, another blood thinner. Second, you should not take more than 1 mg/day of folic acid without medical supervision. Folic acid can interfere with certain laboratory tests and can block the effect of some drugs used to treat epilepsy. Third, if you have kidney failure or are receiving medication for a chronic illness, you should check with your doctor before taking nutritional supplements.

OTHER NUTRITIONAL FACTORS

I have also discussed the importance of proper digestion and assimilation of nutrients. If you do not chew your food thoroughly, or if your digestive system is weak, you may develop nutritional deficiencies, which could adversely affect your bones. A nutrition-oriented doctor can help you determine whether you need to take digestive aids, such as hydrochloric acid, pepsin, or pancreatic enzymes, to improve your absorption of nutrients.

There are theoretical reasons to believe that repeatedly ingesting foods to which you are allergic may promote osteoporosis (discussed in Chapter 17). Identifying and avoiding allergenic foods may not only help relieve many chronic symptoms, it may also help preserve bone mass during your later years.

EFFECTS OF POLLUTION

Studies have suggested that widespread exposure to aluminum may be one of the reasons the incidence of osteoporosis has increased during the past thirty years. In Chapter 19, we discussed the major sources of aluminum in our environment, as well as ways to avoid them. Avoiding aluminum-containing antacids appears to be especially important, since these medications often contain extremely large amounts of aluminum. Chapter 19 also discussed natural ways for you to relieve gastrointestinal problems, so that you would not need antacids. If you do have to take an antacid, Alka-Seltzer or Tums may be preferable, since they contain little or no aluminum.

Exposure to other heavy metals, particularly lead, cadmium, and tin, may also promote osteoporosis. In Chapter 20, simple ways of avoiding these toxic substances were described. The possibility that acid rain contributes to osteoporosis was discussed in Chapter 21.

NATURAL APPROACH TO HORMONE THERAPY

In Chapters 14 through 16, I argued that standard estrogen replacement therapy can be improved upon, both in terms of increased safety and greater effectiveness, by attempting to mimic more closely the natural secretions of the ovary. Where estrogen replacement therapy is concerned, use of the anticarcinogenic estrogen estriol might reduce the cancer risk associated with estrogen treatment. Natural progesterone appears to have a powerful bone-building effect and has been shown to reverse postmenopausal osteoporosis, with virtually no side effects. Preliminary evidence suggests that, in many cases, natural progesterone may be the only hormone needed to prevent or treat osteoporosis, and that estrogen replacement therapy may be necessary only to treat hot flashes, postmenopausal depression, and vaginal atrophy. DHEA, a hormone secreted both by the ovary and the adrenal gland, may also play a role in osteoporosis prevention. In addition, this hormone appears to help prevent cancer, and may be beneficial in the treatment of a wide range of other medical conditions. Judicious use of DHEA, particularly in elderly individuals, may retard or reverse not only osteoporosis but some of the other manifestations of aging as well. In some cases, combining estrogen with testosterone may enhance the effectiveness of estrogen therapy (see Chapter 14).

THE LOGIC OF NATURAL MEDICINE

The most exciting aspect of these new approaches to osteoporosis is that they are, in general, extremely safe. Therefore, even though not all of the answers are in, the potential benefits of these modalities far outweigh the risks. Even if it turns out that the value of this new approach to osteoporosis has been overestimated, taking some of the steps I have recommended may still enhance your health in other ways. Much of what has been discussed in this book falls into the category of "self-care." In other words, you do not need medical supervision to improve your diet, to go on an exercise program, or (with a few exceptions) to take vitamin and mineral supplements. Where hormone replacement therapy is concerned, however, a detailed discussion with an open-minded medical practitioner is necessary.

As is the case in other areas of medicine, the conventional medical community has not yet accepted many of the ideas presented in this book. However, as I argued in Chaper 25, this lack of acceptance is more a result of closed-mindedness and fear among doctors than an indictment of the ideas. The interests of the "medical industry" do not always coincide with the needs of patients, and doctors cannot always be trusted to provide you with the most appropriate, up-to-date information. Fortunately, our society is becoming more aware of the value of nutritional and natural medicine at a time when standard medical care has become too expensive, too dangerous, and too often ineffective.

The evidence presented in this book provides us with a new perspective on osteoporosis. We are finally getting a handle on this modern epidemic. We no longer have to view osteoporosis as a disease with a relentless downhill course. When all of the research is taken into account, bone loss appears to be not only preventable, but reversible, as well. That is good news to the millions of American women who already have osteoporosis and to countless others who are expected to develop it in the future.

With appropriate diet and lifestyle modifications, nutritional supplements, and hormone replacement therapy, millions of fractures may be preventable. It now appears that you have some control over whether or not you will lose your mobility, your independence, or even your life to this dread disease. A new era in the prevention and treatment of osteoporosis is at hand.

Appendix A: Intravenous Vitamin and Mineral Protocol

A description of how I use intravenous vitamins and minerals in my medical practice follows. This information is intended for physicians. Several thousand physicians in the United States are now using this type of treatment in their practice. For many patients, intravenous nutrient therapy is more effective than any other treatment they have tried.

Materials

Magnesium chloride hexahydrate 20%	2–5 cc
Calcium glycerophosphate	2–5 cc
Hydroxocobalamin (1,000 mcg/cc)	1 cc
Pyridoxine hydrochloride (100 mg/cc)	1 cc
Dexpanthenol (250 mg/cc)	1 cc
B-complex 100	1 cc
Vitamin C (222 mg/cc)	1–30 cc

Draw up nutrients into one syringe and inject slowly over 5 to 15 minutes, through a 25G butterfly needle.

PRECAUTIONS

This solution is hypertonic and occasionally causes pain at the site of injection. This can be avoided by diluting the injection 50% with sterile water. Most patients experience warmth during the injection. Too-rapid administration of magnesium can cause a brief period of hypotension, which can be severe. Patients with low blood pressure tend to tolerate less magnesium. When administering this treatment to a patient for the first time, it is best to give 0.5 to 1.0 cc and then wait thirty seconds or so, before proceeding with the rest of the injection. Start with lower doses for elderly or frail individuals.

In patients at risk for hypokalemia, such as those taking certain diuretics, beta-agonists, or corticosteroids, or patients with diarrhea, serum potassium should be measured and hypokalemia should be corrected before administering this treatment. When in doubt, give 20 to 25 mEq of potassium orally at the time of the injection, and repeat 4 to 6 hours later. I have administered more than 10,000 intravenous nutrient injections. When these precautions were followed, I have not seen any serious side effects.

Indications

Chronic fatigue, including
   chronic fatigue syndrome
Chronic depression
Acute or chronic muscle
   spasm; Fibromyalgia
Acute or chronic asthma
Acute or chronic urticaria
   (hives)

Allergic rhinitis
Congestive heart failure
Angina
Ischemic vascular disease
Acute infections
Senile dementia

NOTES

Individuals with severe allergies sometimes react to the preservatives in the injectable products. The most common reactions are headaches, fatigue, or "spaciness." I have not seen a reaction severe enough to require administration of adrenaline. In patients with cardiac arrhythmias, calcium should probably not be included. For asthma or urticaria, 10 to 30 cc of vitamin C and double doses of pyridoxine, dexpanthenol, and vitamin B12 (hydroxocobalamin) may be given.

For infections and allergic rhinitis, 10 to 30 cc of vitamin C are used. In some patients, the treatment works better if vitamin B12 is given intramuscularly in a separate syringe. It is not clear whether this is due to the short half-life of intravenously administered vitamin B12, or whether vitamin B12 interacts with some other component of the injection.

Appendix B: Allergy Elimination Diet and Retesting Program

The following information is used as a teaching guide in my medical practice for identification of food allergies (see Chapter 17 for additional discussion). In general, this type of elimination and retesting program should be done under medical supervision to assure that it is done correctly and to avoid the possibility of nutrient deficiencies from an unbalanced diet.

Foods You Must Avoid

Dairy products milk, cheese, butter, yogurt, sour cream, cottage cheese, whey, casein, sodium caseinate, calcium caseinate, and any food containing these

Wheat most breads, spaghetti, noodles, pasta, most flour, baked goods, durum semolina, and many gravies

Corn including any product with corn oil, vegetable oil from an unspecified source, corn syrup, corn sweetener, dextrose, glucose, corn chips, tortillas, popcorn

Eggs avoid whites and yolks, and any product containing eggs

Citrus Fruits oranges, grapefruits, lemons, limes, tangerines

Coffee, Tea, Alcohol avoid both caffeinated and decaffeinated coffee, as well as standard (such as Lipton) tea and decaffeinated tea; herb teas OK

Refined Sugars including table sugar and any foods that contain it: candy, soda, pies, cake, cookies, and so on. Other names for sugar include sucrose, glucose, dextrose, corn syrup, corn sweetener, fructose, maltose, and levulose. These must all be avoided. Some patients will be allowed 1–3 teaspoons per day of honey or maple syrup. This will be decided on an individual basis.

Honey/Maple Syrup (1–3 teaspoons per day) Allowed ( ) Not allowed ( ).

Food Additives including artificial colors, flavors, preservatives, texturing agents, artificial sweeteners, and so on. Most diet sodas and other dietetic foods contain artificial ingredients and must be avoided.

Any Other Food You Eat More Than Three Times Per Week Any food you are now eating three times per week or more should be eaten no more than every fourth day while on the diet. If you have been eating chicken or iceberg lettuce three or more times a week, avoid them completely and put them in later as test foods. Turkey or other varieties of lettuce may be substituted.

Tap Water (includes cooking water) Allowed ( ) Not allowed ( ).

If tap water is not allowed, use spring or distilled water bottled in glass or heavy plastic. Water bottled in soft (collapsible) plastic tends to leach plastic into the water. Some water filtration systems do not take out all potential allergens.

Note: Many packaged foods contain one or more of these foods. **PLEASE READ LABELS!**

Foods You May Eat

Cereals HOT—oatmeal, oat bran, cream of rye, Rice and Shine; DRY—puffed rice, puffed millet, Oatio's (wheat-free),

Good Shepherd (wheat-free), Crispy Brown Rice Cereal. Diluted apple juice with apple slices and nuts go well on cereal. Soy milk that has no corn oil added (such as some Eden Soy products; please read the ingredients carefully) is OK, also almond nut milk. Most of these foods are available in health food stores.

Grains and Flour Products   rice cakes, rice crackers; Dimplemeyer rye bread (100% rye bread with no wheat); also 100% rye bread from Nature's Garden Bakery; Oriental noodles, such as 100% buckwheat Soba noodles; soy, rice, potato, buckwheat and bean flours; rice or millet bread (as long as they do not contain dairy, eggs, sugar, or wheat); cooked whole grains including oats, millet, barley, buckwheat groats (kasha), rice macaroni, spelt (flour and pasta) brown rice, amaranth, quinoa. Most of these grains are available at health food stores.

Legumes (beans)   including soybeans, tofu, lentils, peas, chickpeas, navy beans, kidney beans, black beans, string beans, and others. Dried beans should be soaked overnight. Pour off the water and rinse before cooking. Canned beans often contain added sugar or other potential allergens. Some cooked beans packaged in glass jars, sold at the health food store, contain no sugar. Read labels. Bean dips without sugar, lemon, or additives are OK. Canned soups include split pea and lentil soup (without additives).

Vegetables   Use a wide variety. All vegetables except corn are permitted.

Proteins   meat, chicken, fish, tuna packed in spring water, turkey, grain or bean casseroles (recipes in vegetarian cookbooks). Shellfish is not restricted from an allergy standpoint, but is not considered particularly healthful. Beef and pork may be eaten unless specified otherwise. Lamb rarely causes allergic reactions, and may be used even when other meats are restricted. Soy cheese may be used as a cheese substitute, if there are no dairy components such as casein or caseinate.

Nuts and Seeds   nuts and seeds, either raw or roasted without salt or sugar. To prevent rancidity, nuts and seeds should be kept in an airtight container in the refrigerator. May also use nut butters from health food stores or from fresh ground nuts (this includes peanut butter, almond butter, cashew butter, walnut butter, sesame butter, and sesame tahini). Nut butters go well on celery sticks and crackers.

Oils and Fats sunflower, safflower, olive, sesame, peanut, flaxseed (edible linseed), and soy oils. Use cold-pressed or expeller-pressed oils (available from health food stores), as they are safer for the heart and blood vessels. Do not use corn oil or "vegetable oil" from an unspecified source, as this is usually corn oil. Also available are Nasoya mayonnaise and Nasoya tofu dressing. Soy and sunflower or safflower margarine are OK from an allergy standpoint, but we do not consider margarine a safe food, as there is evidence it may promote heart disease. It is acceptable to use margarine during the elimination and testing period. However, if you are not allergic to butter we recommend it instead of margarine once you have completed food testing.

Snacks celery, carrot sticks, or other vegetables; fruit in moderation (no citrus); unsalted fresh nuts and seeds; Barbara's Granola Bars (from health food stores); wheat-free cookies (check ingredients). Sweeteners may be honey, barley malt, maple syrup, or fruit juice (not citrus).

Beverages Herb teas (no lemon or orange); spring water in glass bottles; seltzer (salt-free); Perrier; pure fruit juices without sugar or additives (dilute 50:50 with water); almond nut milk (Nut Quick); soy milk without corn oil (such as Eden Soy Plain); Cafix, Inka, and Roma may be used as coffee substitutes.

Tap water contains chlorine, fluoride, and other potentially allergenic chemicals. In some cases, distilled or spring water in glass bottles is the only water allowed. This would include water used for cooking. If tap water is eliminated, it should be reintroduced as if it were a test food. Restrictions on the type of water permitted will be made on a case-by-case basis.

Sweeteners Honey and real maple syrup (not imitation) are allowed in some cases, maximum of 3 teaspoons a day

Thickeners   rice, oat, millet, barley, soy, or amaranth flours; arrowroot, agar

Spices and condiments   salt in moderation, pepper, herbal spices without preservatives or sugar; garlic, ginger, onions; catsup and mustard from the health food store (without sugar); wheat-free tamari sauce; Bragg liquid aminos; vitamin C crystals in water as a substitute for lemon juice

Egg Substitute   (only for use as a binder in baking) Put 1/3 cup water and 1 tablespoon whole flaxseed in small saucepan. Bring to boil, then reduce heat so mixture bubbles slowly. Avoid overheating. Cook five minutes or until mixture is the consistency of a raw egg white. Do not need to strain out flaxseed after cooking. Mixture will bind patties, meat loaves, cookies, and so forth, but will not leaven like eggs for souffles or sponge cakes. Recipe makes enough to substitute for one egg.

Miscellaneous   sugar-free spaghetti sauce; Sorrell Ridge fruit jellies without sugar or lemon juice; other fruit-only jellies that do not contain lemon juice or honey; soups (Hain split pea, lentil, turkey or vegetable, and so on)

Dining Out   Ask for fish topped with slivered almonds without butter or lemon. Get baked potato with a slice of onion on top. Order steak or lamb chops with fresh vegetables. Use salad bars and bring your own dressing (oil and vinegar with chopped nuts or seeds and fresh herbs). At Chinese restaurants, ask for no MSG, corn starch, or soy sauce (contains wheat). Be aware that some other restaurants may also use these ingredients as flavor enhancers.

GENERAL TIPS

Be sure to read labels! Hidden allergens are frequently found in packaged foods. "Flour" usually means wheat; "vegetable oil" may mean corn oil; and casein and whey are dairy products. Make sure your vitamins are free of wheat, corn, sugar, citrus, and so on.

Bioflavonoids in vitamin tablets are usually from citrus. Vary your diet, choosing a wide variety of foods. Do not rely on just a few foods, as you may become allergic to foods you eat every day! **Be sure to eat a good breakfast and have between-meal snacks to prevent your blood sugar from falling while on this diet. If you fail to follow this advice you may lose weight too rapidly on this diet and experience fatigue!** To ensure adequate fiber, eat beans, permitted whole grains, whole fruits and vegetables, nuts and seeds.

WITHDRAWAL SYMPTOMS

About 1 in 4 patients develops mild "withdrawal" symptoms a few days after starting the diet. Withdrawal symptoms may include fatigue, irritability, headaches, malaise, or increased hunger. These symptoms generally disappear within 2 to 5 days and are usually followed by an improvement in your original symptoms. If withdrawal symptoms are too uncomfortable, take vitamin C crystals (from health food stores) 1,000 mg in water, up to four times a day or 3/4 teaspoon of alkali salts (two parts potassium bicarbonate to one part sodium bicarbonate) in water as needed, up to three times a day for several days. Alka Seltzer Gold, two tablets in water, three times a day for several days may also work. Regular Alka Seltzer would also work, but it contains aspirin, which could upset your stomach. In most cases, withdrawal symptoms are not severe and do not require treatment. **It is best to discontinue all of the foods abruptly ("cold turkey"), rather than easing into the diet slowly.**

TESTING INDIVIDUAL FOODS

It may take three weeks for symptoms to improve enough to allow you to retest foods. However, you may begin retesting after two weeks if you are sure you are feeling better. If you have been on the diet for four weeks and feel no better, it is unlikely that food allergies are the cause of your symptoms.

Most patients do improve. Some feel so well on the diet that they decide not to test the foods. This could be a mistake. If you wait too long to retest, your allergies may "settle down" and you will not be able to provoke your symptoms by food testing. Then, you will not know which foods you are allergic to. If reintroducing certain foods causes a recurrence of symptoms, you are probably allergic to those foods.

Allergic reactions to test foods usually occur within ten minutes to twelve hours after ingestion. However, arthritic reactions may be delayed by as much as forty-eight hours. Eat a relatively large amount of each test food (such as a large glass of milk) at breakfast, along with any of the foods on the "permitted" list. If any of your original symptoms come back, or if you develop a headache, bloating, nausea, dizziness, or fatigue, do not eat that food anymore and place it on your "allergic" list. If no symptoms occur, eat the food again for lunch and supper and watch for reactions. Even if the food is well tolerated, do not add it back into your diet until you have finished testing all of the foods. If you are uncertain whether you have reacted to a particular food, remove it from your diet and retest it 4 to 5 days later. Foods you never eat and known offending foods do not have to be tested.

Test Foods in Any Order

Test one new food each day. If your main problem is arthritis, test one new food every other day, since joint pain reactions may be delayed. Test pure sources of a food. Example: do not use pizza to test cheese because pizza also contains wheat and corn oil.

> **Dairy tests** Test milk and cheese on separate days. You may wish to test several cheeses on different days, since some people are allergic to one cheese but not another. It is usually not necessary to test yogurt, cottage cheese, or butter separately.
>
> **Wheat test** Try Wheatena (with no milk or sugar) or another pure wheat cereal. Soy milk may be added.
>
> **Corn test** Use fresh ears of corn or frozen corn (without sauces or preservatives).

Egg test   Test one or two whole eggs, hardboiled, softboiled, or poached, without butter.

Citrus test   Include oranges, grapefruits, lemons, and limes. Test these individually on four separate days. The lemon and lime can be squeezed into Perrier or Seltzer. In the case of orange and grapefruit, use the whole fruit.

Frequently eaten foods   If you have eliminated tap water or any foods that were being consumed more than three times a week, retest them, as well.

Optional Tests

The following foods and beverages are considered undesirable, regardless of whether or not you are allergic to them. If any of them are not now a part of your diet, or if you are fully committed to eliminating them from your diet, there is no need to test them. However, if you have been consuming any of them regularly, it is a good idea to test them and find out how they affect you. Reactions to these foods and beverages may be severe in some cases. They should be tested only on days that you can afford to feel bad.

Coffee and tea tests (separate days)   Do not add milk, non-dairy creamer, or sugar. You may add soy milk. If you use decaffeinated coffee, test it separately. Coffee, tea, decaffeinated coffee, and decaffeinated tea are separate tests.

Sugar test   Put 4 teaspoons of sugar in a drink or on cereal, or mix it with another food.

Chocolate test   Use 1 to 2 tablespoons of pure baker's chocolate or Hershey's cocoa powder.

Alcohol test (test this last)   Beer, wine, and hard liquor may require testing on different days, as the reactions to each may be different. Have two drinks per test day, but only if you can afford not to feel well that day and possibly the next day.

Food additive test   Buy a set of McCormick's or French's food dyes and colors. Put 1/2 teaspoon of each color in a glass. Add one teaspoon of the mixture to a glass of pineapple juice or diluted (50:50 with water) grape juice.

Rotation Diets

At your follow-up visit, you may need to discuss rotation diets. One cause of food allergy is eating the same foods all of the time. If you have an allergic constitution and eat the same foods every day, you may eventually become allergic to them. After you have discovered which foods you can eat safely, make an attempt to rotate your diet. A four-day schedule is necessary for some severely allergic patients, but most people can tolerate foods more frequently than every four days. Use common sense and consume a wide variety of foods. Do not just latch onto a few favorites. **It is not necessary to do strict food rotation during the elimination and retesting periods.**

ADDITIONAL INFORMATION: SYMPTOMS THAT MAY BE DUE TO FOOD ALLERGY

General fatigue, anxiety, depression, insomnia, food cravings, obesity

Infections recurrent colds, urinary tract infections, sore throats, ear infections, yeast infections

Ear, Nose, and Throat chronic nasal congestion, postnasal drip, fluid in the ears, Menière's syndrome

Gastrointestinal irritable bowel syndrome, constipation, diarrhea, abdominal cramping, ulcerative colitis, Crohn's disease, gallbladder disease

Cardiovascular high blood pressure, arrhythmia, angina

Dermatologic acne, eczema, psoriasis, canker sores (aphthous ulcers), hives

Rheumatologic muscle aches, osteoarthritis, rheumatoid arthritis

Neurologic migraines and other headaches, numbness

Miscellaneous   asthma, frequent urination, teeth grinding, bedwetting, infantile colic

Note: Most of these disorders have more than one cause, but food allergy is a relatively common and frequently overlooked cause.

Index